From Fat to Fit in 1 Year:

How
I
Defeated
Obesity
Forever

A 28 kg/62 lb demonstrable weight loss achievement

Jorge Zuazola ©

ISBN-13: 978- 1468073706 ISBN-10: 1468073702

DEDICATION

This book is entirely dedicated to my daughter Carmen to whom I would like to say:

1. I was wrong

2. I am sorry

3. You can do it

4. I believe in you

5. I am proud of you

6. Thank you

7. I need you

8. I trust you

9. I respect you

10. I love you

INDEX

FORMAT AND BOOK DUPLICATION VIA LINKEDIN

This book is defined with a best seller because it relies on unique concepts such as:
• Leadership
• Network
• Duplication
• LinkedIn

All members "know" themselves via LinkedIn's, the largest network of professionals with over 100 million users. LinkedIn is a company who went public in May 2011 in the United States. It is therefore relevant to explain the structure of this book as it has 100 pages of A4 size which would be between 250-300 pages of a normal book. This book is thus a leader which thrives on the strength of its network to double.

Format

The format is designed so that the reader can get the most personal growth of himself.

Often many best-selling books are about 250 pages of text and much smaller than this.

This causes in many occasions that the reader forgets the content learned in the book. In this case the reader can look at the self-empowering blog in Appendix II designed to make the most out of the book.

The function of leadership is not to create more followers but to create more leaders. The successful duplication of leaders depends on the success of a great leader. Therefore, this book is born with the vocation of a leader who seeks to empower people to learn the concepts explained here.

This book consists of

• A detailed Index to chapter and section so that the reader can always refer to any book page.

• A corporate manual style format for the reader to use the book in their professional and daily life to apply the concepts.

• A blank blog at the end to take notes and leadership quotes and use Twitter and LinkedIn in order to increase your personal brand value in the market.

Duplication LinkedIn

The power of duplication is unlimited. But people do not know it. If you were offered a million Euros on June 1, 2011 v a cent of a Euro doubling it self only 30 days, you should know that the cent is better because you actually lose more than 4 million Euros if you ignore the duplication. Below the test statistics based on the contact section of the founder of Spanish LinkedIn Leadership. This tells you the duplication of his LinkedIn network.

Here you see statistics about your network, including how many users you can reach through your connections. Your network grows every time you add a connection — **Invite connections now**.

Your Network of Trusted Professionals

You are at the center of your network. Your connections can introduce you to 17,067,500+ professionals — here's how your network breaks down:

Your Connections   <u>3,260</u>
Your trusted friends and colleagues

Two degrees away   2,056,500+
Friends of friends; each connected to one of your connections

Three degrees away   15,007,700+
Reach these users through a friend and one of their friends

Total users you can contact through an Introduction   17,067,500+

22,512 new people in your network since December 6

The LinkedIn Network

The total of all LinkedIn users, who can be contacted directly through InMail. Total users you can contact directly — **try a search now!**
135,000,000+

More About Your Network

REGIONAL ACCESS *Top locations in your network:*

5%
1. Greater New York City Area

4%
2. San Francisco Bay Area

3%
3. London, United Kingdom

2%
4. Greater Chicago Area

2%
5. Greater Los Angeles Area

Your region: Frankfurt Am Main Area, Germany

Your connections are in 420 locations but your network gives you access to **2,623 additional locations**, including:

- Gurgaon, India
- Ahmedabad Area, India
- Rochester, New York Area

Fastest growing locations in your network:

1. Madrid Area, Spain
2. Barcelona Area, Spain
3. Paris Area, France

INDUSTRY ACCESS *Top industries in your network:*

1. Information Technology and Services — 12%

2. Marketing and Advertising — 5%

3. Computer Software — 5%

4. Financial Services — 5%

5. Human Resources — 4%

Your industry: Consumer Goods

Your connections are in 125 industries but your network gives you access to **148 additional industries**, including:

- Gambling & Casinos
- Photography
- Medical Practice

Fastest growing industries in your network:

1. Information Technology and Services
2. Consumer Goods
3. Marketing and Advertising

In conclusion, this book has the makings of a best seller. It is marketed in all the book distribution websites in the world. But the vocation of duplication in LinkedIn, which integrates Twitter, is the key to its success in its strategic goal of becoming a best seller.

CHAPTER 1. Leadership is about people from beginning to end: Learn to be a leader through teamwork and sports

"Sports is a school for life"

- Vicente del Bosque

I am the founder of www.spanisleadership.com . We define leadership in a single sentence

Leadership is all about people from beginning to an end

Most Spanish people (and people around the world) would wrongly say that leadership is vision, courage, credibility, determination or even militarism or politics. At Spanish Leadership we however sincerely believe that leadership is first and foremost about people. It is about leaders releasing people to do what they need to do in the most productive and beneficial way. You cannot call yourself a leader and not have followers.

A leader's greatest compliment and achievement is his or her followers, and followers will reflect a leader's positive value and missions. Logically the opposite is also true. Flawed leadership – for example, the lack of integrity that, sadly, we so often associate with today's Spain based politicians- will also reproduce itself in followers.

That is why Spanish Leadership's motto is TEAM which stands for

Together

Everybody

Achieves

More.

That is why we feature only our sportsmen in our website. We are proud of them Spanish Leadership is an English speaking treble iii (Internet Ideas Incubator). It has to be in English because sadly most of our countrymen and women think that being fluent in English is not a must. They wrongly believe that someone will come to put them a red carpet to become proficient in English. All the members of Spanish leadership are native Spanish speakers. However, as a team, we bring to the table over a century of international experience in Europe, US, Asia Pacific, Africa and South America. We are all proficient in English.

Leadership is just about taking action and motivating others to do the same. Contrary to widespread belief, leadership is not just about holding a position or spouting what you believe. Most people do not understand (or do not want to understand) that positions and job titles come and go. Actions and relationships are the marks of true leadership, and they last forever.

Without people there can never be leadership. People are the heart, soul and spirit of any organization. Without them there is no need for leaders. Leaders are therefore responsible to see people use their assets. They are the ones responsible for the next generation of leadership.

A picture is worth more than 1.000 words:

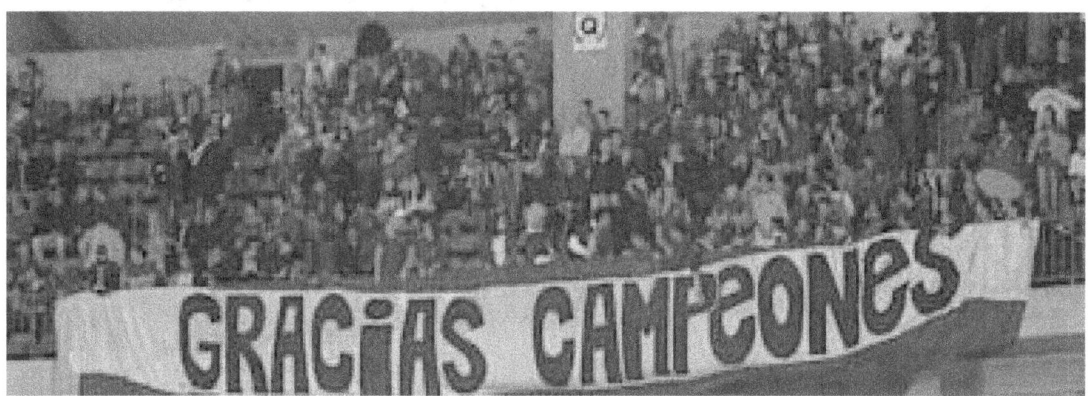

This picture, together with the banner on the Spanish flag with the motto **"Gracias Campeones/Thank you Champions",** taken at the Brussels King Baldouin Stadium during the 2010 World Cup game between Belgium and Spain, is a true example of people´s leadership. 12.000 Spaniards of Belgium, Holland, France, Germany and the UK showed up at the stadium to continue with the relationship with the national team. Whereas the game was not critical, it did not matter to the Spaniards. **Leadership is all about people and we all wanted to be there in the first game in a key European city after the success in Vienna where Spain clinched the European title after 44 years. 15.000 in Vienna and 12.000 in Brussels mean leadership.** When I mentioned to Xavi Hernández (Euro 2008´s most valued player) in our occasional encounter at Brussels´Zaventum airport (see picture below)

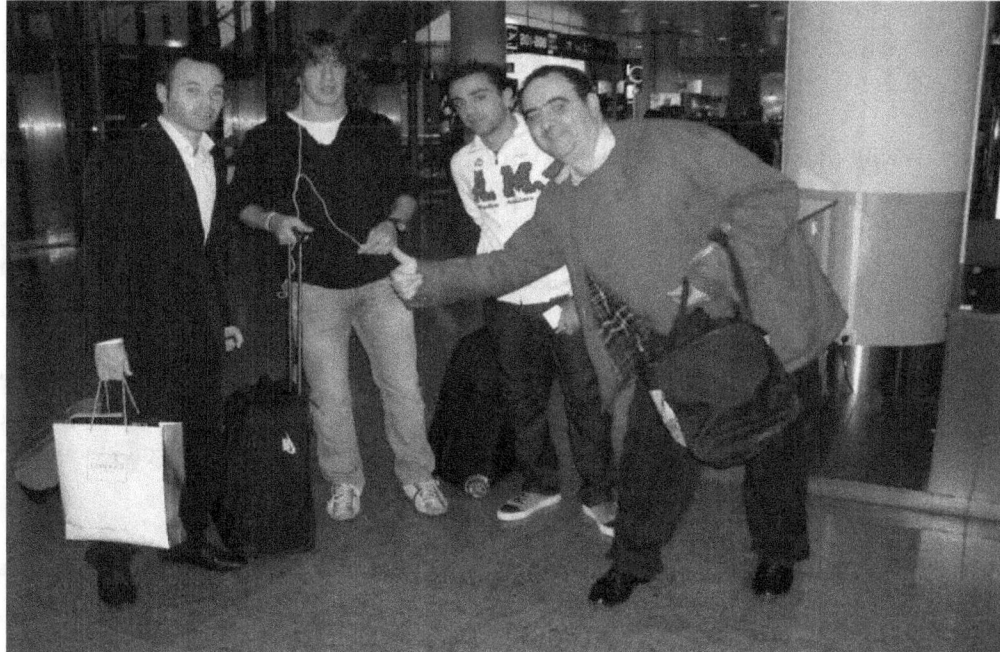

that the above banner had inspired me so much as to create something called spanishleadership.com, he told me : "Really"? "Definitely" I said. "Don't you think that 12.000 Spaniards from 5 leading European countries would not come all the way to Brussels on a Wednesday night if we did not believe in your leadership"? I asked. Xavi nodded.

The old tag of underachievers , which many tabloids in Britain used to attribute to the Spanish national team, is no longer there. It is irrelevant if we get knocked out soon in the World Cup. The question which comes to mind is whether or not the underachievers tag ever existed. If we look at the natural progression of Fernando Torres until he became European Champion scoring the winning goal, it would appear the underachievers tag never existed in the first place.

1.1. Fernando Torres career: leadership from beginning to end

Generally speaking media perceptions tend to be wrong. In the case of Spanish football the underachievers tag perception was always incorrect.

Because of the relevance of the Premier League world-wide and the fact that Fernando Torres was the goal scorer in the Euro 2008 final, the media perception is now that Torres ended the underachievers tag on 29th June 2008 at the Ernst Happel Stadium in Vienna.

But the perception is once again wrong.

Fernando Torres has always been an example of Spanish leadership as evidenced by the following:

- Born in the outskirts of the Spanish capital Madrid, he joined Atlético Madrid´s football club **with just 10 years of age.**

- Prior to reaching the Spanish Premier League he played in the Spanish second division with his club. To achieve promotion he had to endure 2 seasons in the second division.

- During those years in the second division (2001 and 2002) Fernando Torres was however awarded two unique distinctions every year. In both 2001 and 2002 he was nominated top scorer and best player of both the UEFA Under 16 (2001) and Under 19 (2002) European Championships. That is **4 distinctions over 2 years for a second division player.**

- Prior to becoming European Champion at senior level in 2008, Fernando Torres had already been Euro Champion at junior level twice and had also defeated the all-mighty Germany in those tournaments. His goal against Germany in the Euro 2008 was therefore not a surprise but a repetition of previous performances.

- In a total of 287 games since he started his career with Atlético Madrid to the end of his first season in England, Fernando Torres scored 124 goals in all competitions which is indeed an outstanding record because it includes the first two seasons (43 games) in the second division where he had the handicap of either not being a regular player or not scoring enough goals.

SUMMARY OF FERNANDO TORRES´NUMBERS

Club	Season	League		FA Cup		UEFA/Champions League		Total	
		Games	Goals	Games	Goals	Games	Goals	Games	Goals
Atlético de Madrid	2000–01*	4	1	2	0			6	1
	2001–02*	36	6	1	1			37	7
	2002–03	29	13	2	1			31	14
	2003–04	35	19	5	2			40	21
	2004–05	38	16	6	2	5	2	49	20
	2005–06	36	13	4	0			40	13
	2006–07	36	14	4	1			40	15
	Total	**214**	**82**	**24**	**7**	**5**	**2**	**243**	**91**
Liverpool FC	2007–08	33	24	1	3	10	6	44	33
Total		**247**	**106**	**25**	**10**	**15**	**8**	**287**	**124**

*Second division

Title	Team	Country	Year
UEFA Under 16 Euro Champs	Spain	England	2001
UEFA Under 19 Euro Champs http://es.wikipedia.org/wiki/Campeonato_Europeo_de_la_UEFA_Sub-19	Spain	Norway	2002
UEFA Euro 2008	Spain	Austria	2008

Award	Year
Top scorer UEFA Under 16 Euro Champs	2001
Best player UEFA Under 16 Euro Champs	2001
Top scorer UEFA Under 19 Euro Champs	2002
Best player UEFA Under 19 Euro Champs	2002

| Best Premier League rookie | 2008 |
| Best player of the final game in Euro 2008 | 2008 |

And yet despite the above examples, it is not clear that Torres is a better striker than Villa. In fact it looks like the other way round, Villa´s numbers in the Spanish premier league and the national team, outweigh those of Torres. Therefore this is a true example of Spanish leadership once again: if Fernando Torres has been able to achieve all the numbers of the enclosed table, the question which comes to mind is: how much can Villa deliver? The answer is that probably much more.

1.2.   Fernando Torres links up and networks with people

In the morning of 29th June 2008, at the Hilton Plaza Hotel in Vienna, Austria, the Spanish coach Luis Aragonés gave a kiss to Fernando Torres after the mentoring chat in the hotel. The kiss was justified: Aragonés coached Torres while he was a teenager in the second division. He made him a man in football terms. Fernando had already reached maturity during his outstanding first season at Liverpool.

However David Villa was injured. The coach knew that Torres was the only chance to score given that our top goal scorer would not play the final. Therefore he showed his affection.

When the players were coming down from the hotel room to the bus (see picture below) I told all of them Gracias (thank you in Spanish). Yet when Torres passed by I spoke to him in English and said "Fernando the whole world is watching you today". He looked back and smiled before getting into the bus whose motto was "Whatever happens Spain forever"

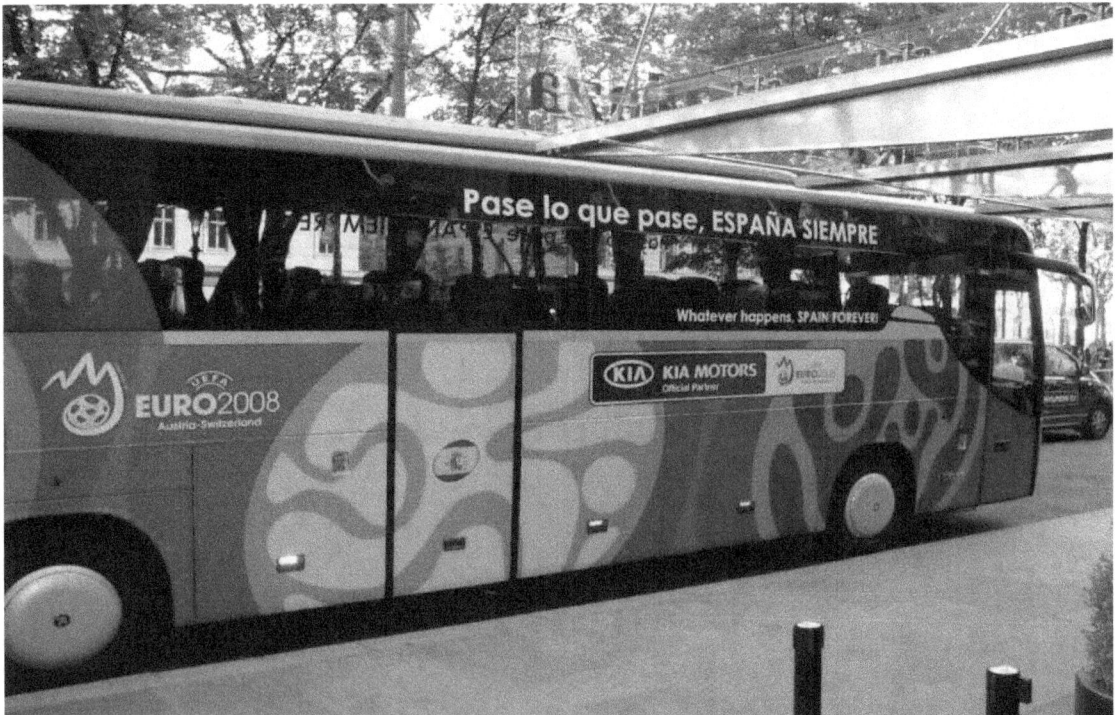

2 years later, on March 3rd I had the opportunity to rejoin with Fernando. This time in París, France.

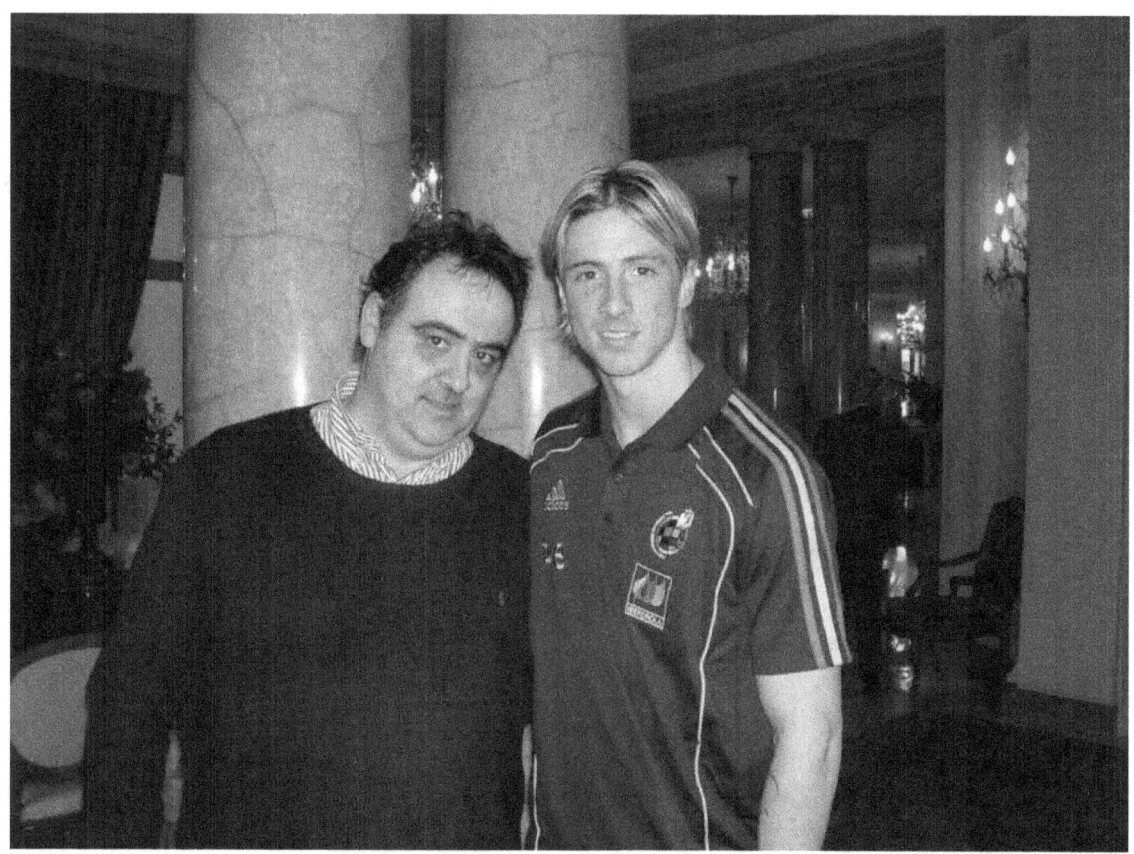

1.3.   My encounter with Fernando Torres put my change strategy in motion

When I was about to publish my first leadership book end of April 2010, I saw that Fernando Torres, Steven Gerrard (http://uk.linkedin.com/pub/steven-gerrard/3/11a/236) had just opened a LinkedIn account and Cristiano Ronaldo (http://es.linkedin.com/in/cristianoronaldo) had been told to put his career with Real Madrid in his profile. They are all in the same network that I use daily namely www.linkedin.com

I have taken the spots example in the first chapter of this book to inspire the reader with the title and concept of about linking up and networking with people. Sports management is the leading example of the concept of TEAM

Together
Everybody
Achieves
More

You need to make this mental shift i.e. the successful running of companies (whether large or small) depends on the TEAM, network and linked up concepts for the next decade.

I then realized that most of my setbacks in life did come out of one single problem: obesity. In subsequent chapters I will refer to this. Obesity is an illness. The root cause of it is ignorance.

I realized that the dream of being with Fernando and his team mates in Johannesburg on July 11th 2010 to see them clinching gold again for the second time in a row, could only be achieved through sports discipline.

The person who took the picture of us is Diario AS´s International Director, my dear friend Joaquin Maroto. He laughed at my weight. When 2 months later in May I told him that I was about to do my daily jogging session he laughed over the phone: "You ? You cannot run, can You ?. "

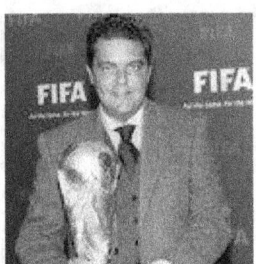

Joaquín Maroto
@AS_Maroto

Joaquín was right but he missed one point. When a man has a dream he cannot be denied. Earlier in the year, in April 2010, I had revisited my 6 original non-negotiable dreams to add a further 21 dreams. One of this additional dreams was to see Spain lifting the World Cup trophy life in a football stadium. Like most people I forgot that I wrote the dream down. I rediscovered it in September 2010 some 2 months after the World Cup.

I did then realize that what set me in motion to start obesity were three clear cut mental concepts:

a) Leadership is all about people
b) Sports and teamwork go hand in hand
c) Dreams do come true provided they are in writing because a dream is a goal with a deadline

I said to myself that by March 2011 I did want to look a complete different person. It was exactly a year later after Joaquin took my picture with the famous Fernando Torres.

Now my friend Joaquin cracks jokes at me saying: "Before you need Andoni Goikoetxea´s national T-shirt but now you are so slim that you can wear that of Jesús Navas our slim right wing forward"

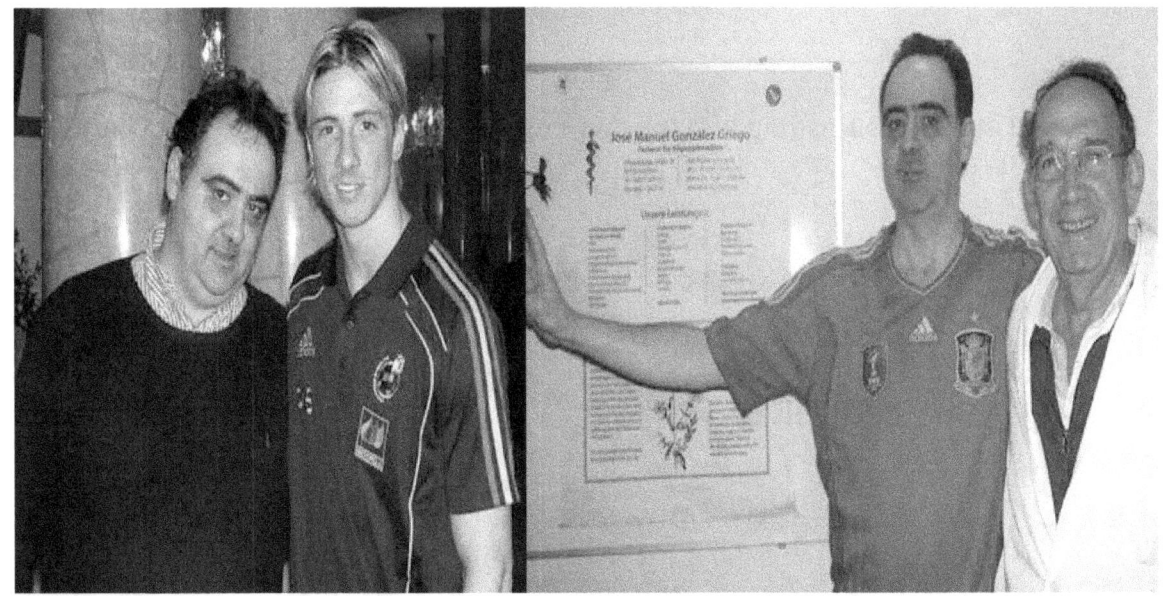

A picture is always worth more than 1000 words, isn´t it ? The difference is 28 kg on the spot: 108.5 kg in March 2010. 80.5 kg in March 2011. 28 kg equate to 62 lb

CHAPTER 2.Reading is to the mind what food is to the body

"In defeat I discovered the head and tail of the same coin but my inner reading was the experience I gained with it"

- Arantxa Sánchez-Vicario

"I have never known any distress that an hour´s reading did not relieve"

- Montesquieu

"You are going to have negative poison dumped into to your mind and emotions every day of your life by TV; newspapers and people. Therefore listen to a few minutes of positive material before you start the day and then read. Leaders are readers."

-Zig Ziglar

2.1   The first hour is the rudder of the day. That is your golden hour.

It has taken me from 1998 when I first heard this in the CD to 2011 to fully apply it. The first hour of the day is your golden hour because it is the rudder of the day. The secret is to wake up 1 hour earlier than you do now. Spend that hour on your own reading. Do not blame family or circumstances. Prepare yourself mentally for the challenges of the day.

As you will see in section 2.2 I did read 3 books a month many months of 2010 when I took the decision to defeat obesity. Yet until January 2011 I have not adhered to the golden hour rule.

It is a matter of habits.

We first have to form the champions habits. Once we have those habits, we become people of success.

My daily schedule starts now at 5 am. From 5 to 6 I listen to a CD and read a book. Then I go to the swimming pool after taking my nutrition bar. At 7.30 I have a normal breakfast and start getting productive at 8 am. But to achieve this perfect control of my mind and time I had to read monthly and put goals in writing. This is how I did it.

2.2   The discipline of daily reading and the subsequent loss weight each month

	Book read	Author	Month/Weight	Inspirational quotes and sentences
1.	Your roadmap for success: You can get there from here.	John C. Maxwell	March 2010 108.5 kg	Success is not measured by what a man accomplishes, but by the opposition he has encountered, and the courage with which he has maintained the struggle against overwhelming odds (Aviator Charles Lindbergh) For every negative remark to a family member, it takes 4 positive statements to counteract the damage. (John C. Maxwell) Sustain a family life for a long period of time and you can sustain success for a long period of time. First things first. If you life is in order you can do whatever you want. (NBA coach Pat Riley) Many people dream of success. To me success can be achieved only through repeated failure and instrospection. In fact, success only represents 1 percent of your work that results from 90 percent of that which is called failure. Very few unacquainted with failure will ever know the true joy of success (Sochiro Honda) I will go even farther and say that no person unacquainted with failure will know success (John C. Maxwell) Nothing in the world can take the place of persistence. Talent will not ; nothing is more common than unsuccessful men with talent. Genius will not ;

			unrewarded genius is almost a proverb. Education will not ; the world is full of educated derelicts. Persistence and determination aloner are omnipotent (President Calvin Coolidge, quote also used by McDonald's founder Ray Kroc)
2. Attitude is everything	Jeff Keller	March 2010 107.8 kg	To change your circumstances, first start thinking differently (Normant Vincent Peale)
3. The purpose driven life: What on earth I am here for?	Rick Warren	March 2010 106.5 kg	If you don't have any Bible verses memorized, you've got no bullets in your gun ! I challenge you to memorize one verse a week for the rest of your life. Imagine how much stronger you will be.
4. Acres of Diamond	Russell H. Conwell	April 2010 106 kg	Money is power. You have to be reasonable ambitious to have it ! You can do more good things with it than without it. Money printed the Bible, built its churches, send messengers and pay the priests, there would not be many of them if they were not paid. But I know there are more important things than money and more worth than gold. Love (Carmen) is the greatest thing of God's creation. Yet bless the lover (me as father I have to) who has a lot of money.
5. El ser excelente (2nd reading)	Miguel Angel Cornejo	April 2010 105 kg	The excellent human being is the one who does the things not the one who looks for reasons for not doing them. JUST DO IT
6. Becoming a resonant leader	Annie McKee Richard Boyatzis Frances Johnston	April 2010 104 kg	The authors conclude and explain that many of the leaders they have studied (mainly Coporate World) get caught in the Sacrifice Syndrome. But they also show how leaders can adopt this syndrome when they adopt practises and spark renewal : mindfulness, hope and comparison. By taping into mindfulness and cultivating the capacity for hope and compassion, leaders manage the

				cycle of sacrifice and renewal while sustaining resonance and effectiveness over time.
7.	177 Mental toughness secrets of the World Class	Steve Siebold	May 2010 103.5 kg	**It is the middle class the one which is more incongruent with reality. The working class just concentrates on surviving. The middle class trades time more for money. However the world-class trades ideas that solve problem for money. Money flows from ideas like water.**
8.	Adding the "E" to your business strategy	Lars Hilse	May 2010 103 kg	Take your time and digest what you have read. Since you have ignored the Internet for the last 15 years anyhow, another few months are unlikely to put you out of business. Regardless if you are an entepreneur or have an existing business that you are looking to expand : if you utilize these and similar measures you can easliy increase business by : -generating leads - increasing the visibility of your venture - boosting the value of your operation As you have probably figured while reading it is very important to find the right combination between the instruments in order to get most out of them
9.	Focal Point: A proven system to simplify your life, double your productivity and achieve all your goals	Brian Tracy	May 2010 102.5 kg	By setting goals and priorities, and by focusing on higher-value activities anyone can increase his or her overall productivity and performance by 1/1000 over the next 24 hours. Many people could double or triple their overall productivity in the next 24 hours if they really wanted to. If you continually learn, study and upgrade your skills, clarify and reclarify your goals, set

			better and clearer priorities, and focus on progressively more valuable tasks, you can increase your overall productivity performance and output by 0.1% each day, day after day, indefinitely. If you become 0.1% more productive each day, five days per week, at the end of a week you will be 0.5 percent more productive. At the end of 4 weeks, you will be 2% more productive (4 x 0.25). At the end of 52 weeks (52/4=13) you will be 26% more productive (i.e. 2 x 13 =26)
10. Emotional Intelligence	Daniel Goleman	June 2010 102 kg	Emotions have no place in intelligence and only muddle picture of mental life In the day-to-day world no intelligence is more importan than the interpersonal
11. How to Think Like a CEO and Act Like a Leader	Michael F. Andrew	June 2010 101.5 kg	90 % of success is showing up
12. 150 Bible Verses Every Catholic Should Know	Patrick Madrid	June 2010 101 kg	**Humility is the queen of virtues as long as you memorize it and repeat it at all times** **John 16 :33 « I have said this to you, that in me you may have peace. In the world you have tribulation;but be of good cheeer, I have overcome the world »** What a marvelous verse to commit to memory and ponder in your heart, each and every day or your life ! No doubt you will experience troubles : illness, financial setbacks, strife, confrontations, loneliness. Life is difficult ; there is no way around it. But keep your eyes fixed on Jesus ; and these troubles will pale to insignificance. They are passing away soon to be forgotten.
13. Rhinoceros Success	Scott Alexander	June 2010 101 kg	Positive thinking will get you nothing unless you combine it

			with charging. Talking is only an oral exercise, unless you ACT on what you say. Dreams are only dreams, unless you become a rhinoceros and charge at them.
14. No Excuses-The Power of Self-Discipline	Brian Tracy	July 2010 100.5 kg	Out of 1000 success principles which one is the most important ? – **"Self-discipline which is the ability to do what you should do, when you should do it, whether you feel like it or not. There are 999 other success principles that I have found in my reading and experience, but without self-disciplined, none of them work. With self-discipline, they all work"**
15. Stress for Success	Jim Loehr	July 2010 100 kg	It all comes down to a method of acting: The best performers are invariably the best actors and actresses. What possible connection is there between issues of IPS, productivity, emotional intelligence and the notion of acting ? The answer is EVERYTHING. If you review a situation in which highlight trained professional actors are instructed to portray anger and compare it with situations in which actors become genuinely angry, when their emotion is real not faked, you will find that the difference is NOTHING. They are indistinguishable because once the amygdala is turned on, the physiology follows. And when physiology is activated, the emotion becomes real. **Without question, the tools professional actors are using to summon emotions called for in their scripts could have powerful applications in the real world. The best ISP example is the tennis player Chris Evert.** She was a superb actress and could

			summon IPS almost at will. Anyone who hopes to be a star in the corporate arena can benefit from studying her career. She learned a unique response to the same conditions that were destroying her competitors: she thrived on the conditions of competitions (i.e. she grew herself up in the conditions of competitions). If a call went against her or she hit a bad shot at a crucial moment, she went about her business in her controlled, cool way, letting nothing ruffle her. As skilled actress, her every action on the court evidenced remarkable emotional intelligence
16. Jonathan Livingston Seagull: A story	Richard Bach	July 2010 100 kg	Irresponsibility does not pay. Life is the unknown and the unknowable, except that we are put into this world to eat, to stay alive as long as we possibly can. Boredom and fear and anger are the reasons that a gulf´s life is so short, and with these gone from his thought, he lived a long fine life indeed Your whole body from wingtip to wingtip is no more than your thought itself, in a form you can see. Break the chains of your thought, and you break the chains of your body too…
17. Grow up: How taking responsibility can make you a happy adult	Dr. Frank Pittman	August 2010 100 kg	Dr. Pittman quite implicitly admits that anti-depressants do not work because he says " If your brain is chemically unable to slip into happiness even 1. after you have stopped drinking 2. started getting exercising daily 3. conquered your anger 4. revealed all your secret shames,

24

			5. stopped the behavior that made you feel guilty, 6. became more loving to everyone they were to you, 7. taken up a full complement of work and play, and 8. learned how to be a grown-up and practiced it, then you may benefit from antidepressants. And he adds "but do all the other things first, before you start blaming your genes" which….really means If you do 1 to 8 above then anti-depressants are not necessary
18. Choice Theory: A new psychology of personal freedom	William Glaser	August 2010 100 kg	The Spanish word **ganas** describes the strong desire to engage in this struggle better than any word I know. It means the desire to work hard, carry on, do whatever it takes to ensure survival, and go beyond survival to security. **Ganas** is a highly valuable trait; if you want a job done, hire someone with a lot of it. If you are looking for a mate you can count on to help build a family and a life with you, find one with **ganas** and treat him or her well. Try not to criticize this motivated mate; you don´t want the **ganas** turned against you.
19. What they don´t teach you at Harvard Business School	Mark. H. McCormack	August 2010 100 kg	Acting rather than reacting allows you to use what you have learnt Acting allows you to convert perceptions into controls By reacting, by failing to step back first, you are probably throwing away the advantage of acting. If you don´t react you will never over-react. You will be the controller rather than the controlled Street smart-thinking gives you a slight pyschological edge over others Street smart-thinking helps you to get the most ouf of the others Street smart-thinking is an applied people sense Running a company is a constant process of breaking out of systems and challenging conditioned reflexes

			Running a company is a constant process of rubbing against the grain
			Learn to be a good listener
			Aggresive observation does not mean hasty observation but
			Converting signals into usable perceptions
20. The Secret Language of Leadership: How leaders inspire action through narrative	Stephen Denning	September 2010 99 kg	The language of leadership has its own grammar. Just as in the English language and adjective comes before its noun, and the subject generally comes before the verb, the language of leadership requires that getting attention comes before anything else, and that stimulating desire for change becomes before providing reasons for change. Why is this so ? It is a function of the way human beings are structured. Underlying psychological mechanisms make these patterns and sequences more resonant than others. Ultimately the implication of the language of leadership is this : there is a pattern of simple narratives that, under the right enabling conditions, will make any worthwhile change idea difficult to resist. The task of leadership is to find it.
21. How I raised myself from failure to success in selling	Frank Bettger	September 2010 98.5 kg	« My great concern is not whether or not you have failed, but whether you are content with your failure » (Abraham Lincoln). Thomas Edison had 10.000 failures before he invented the incandescent bulb. Edison made up his mind that each failure brought him that much closer to success. Nobody will remember the times you struck out in the early innings if you hit a home run with the bases full in the ninth. Failure means nothing at all if success comes eventually. And that is a thought that should cheer you and help you keep on keeping on when the going seems hard. Keep going ! Each week, each

			month, you are improving. One day soon, you will find a way to do the thing that today looks impossible. It was Shakespeare who wrote « Our doubts are traitors, and make us lose the good we oft might win, by fearing to attempt » **Courage is not the absence of fear, it is the conquest of it.**
22. Copy Cat Marketing 101	Burke Hedges	September 2010 98 kg	Network marketing is the ultimate synergism because it combines the best from the concept of franchising…with the best from the concept of exponential growth. It is a marriage made in heaven ! If we see a great movie, like Forrest Gump, we recommend it to our friends. But we do not get paid when our friends go to see it ? NO, of course not. Same goes for recommending a great restaurant. We tell our friends and family when we eat at a terrific restaurant – but does the owner give us a commision on our friends´dinner tab ? NO WAY ! In Network Marketing, you get paid a commission for recommending products and services that you use and recommend anyway. It is a win/win situation – and it is the most effective, most ethical kind of marketing in the world.
23. Network marketing: A way of life	Janusz Szajna	October 2010 97 kg	In his book Promises To Keep Charles Paul Conn reminds us an old Hindu story about four blind men. Each one of them touched an elephant, and was supposed to tell others what the elephant was. One man touched the tail, the second touched a leg, the third touched the belly, and the fourth man tapped the side. A discussion followed, even a quarrel, about nature of

			this thing called the elephant. Each man was convinced that he was right.

When people talk about network maketing, they base their opinion on what they have personally experienced in network marketing. Everybody thinks his information is only true one, and shares his experience with others. People I meet most often are the ones who had a short, accidental contact, with MLM ; poked it with a stick a few years before. They remember their impressions, and add colors to their memories. |
| 24. What to say when you talk to yourself (4th reading) | Shad Helmstetter | October 2010 96 kg | What adults tell us as children has an incredibly important effect on us. It forms what we believe about most of what is going on around us and almost everything that we come to believe about ourselves.

You can reprogram. You can erase the old negative counter-productive, work against you, programming and replace it with a healthy, new, positive, productive kind of programming. **And it is easy. Erase and replace. All you have to do is to learn how to talk to yourself.**

If we change our attitudes and our behaviour just by changing our programming, then none of us have to continue struggling through life then none of us have to continue struggling with our old, negative programming dragging us down or holding us back. If we can just learn to give specific, productive new directions to our minds, then we have a chance to make things work – and keep working. |

| 25. The Power of Talking Out Loud to Yourself (2nd reading) | Bill Wayne | October 2010 95 kg | When you talk out loud to yourself, you can cause yourself to focus intently on the challenge, situation or circumstance. This activity increases the likelihood of obtaning a desirable solution more quickly. It is easy to daydream nonproductively for an hour or two, but it only wastes time and doesn´t give you the results you would like to have. It is incredibly powerful hearing your own voice emotionally proclaiming what you intent and expect to accomplish. Talking out loud to yourself can go a long way in helping you.

Those who pursue their dreams are often thought of as being crazy- generally by those who aren´t moving on. But don´t concern yourself with that. It is their problem, not yours. This is your life, and you have the right to go after your dreams with all your might. Now let us get on with it. |
| 26. How to stop worrying and start living | Dale Carnegie | November 2010 88 kg | Our life is what our thoughts make it

Think and act cheerfully and you will feel cheerful

When we hate our enemies we are giving them power over us, power over our
• Sleep
• Appetites
• Blood Pressure
• Health &
• Happiness

When Jesus said « Love your enemies » he was not only preaching sound ethics. He was also preaching tweentieth-century medicine. When He |

			said « Forgive 77 times » Jesus was telling you and me how to keep from having high blood pressure, heart trouble, stomach ulcers and many other ailments.
27. The Winning Way to Success! How to Win in Life and Enjoy the Journey	Ronnie Kagan	December 2010 87 kg	One good idea is all you need to birth a fortune GOSPA Model = Goal Objectives Strategies Planning Analysis SMART = Specific Measurable Aligned Realistic Time Bound
28. Secrets of closing the sale	Zig Ziglar	December 2010 86 kg	Stand up, put your hands on your shoulders and sweep away that little sales killing devil who is whispering in your ears Calls produce sales and no calls produce no sales Psychology = common sense if you want to be a truly professional person Women have developed instinct or intuition to a much finer point than men If your qualification process or presentation is weak, you are not going to be able to pressure many people in our sophisticated society There is no such a thing as a good salesman who is poor closer Selling without closing is like lathering without saving Little things determine sales results Too early close is when you attempt to close the sale before establishing in the prospect´s mind value for what you sell Closing a deal (sale) means you have converted invested time into a profitable time
29. The Optimal Health Revolution	Dr Duke Johnson	January 2011 84 kg	A revolution starts with a fundamental change in what we think. It starts with a new way of understanding the world. Understanding becomes belief. And belief changes the way we live and behave for the rest of our lives. The revolution starts with you – with taking responsibility for your own health. Not that you haven´t

			wanted to. If you are like most people you just haven´t understood what to do. The result: Your thinking, your beliefs, and your lifestyle are leading you down the path to premature death from chronic diseases. The way to optimal health and longevity involves broad lifestyle changes. It is real revolution, not a phony quick fix. If you join this revolution, you will lose weight – assuming your excessive body fat to start with. But you will use it as a result of achieving a healthy lifestyle, not the other way around. Losing weight will be a healthy side effect of reducing your risk of chronic disease and early death. (Rafael Blanco Elgert, every kilogram you lose, an additional year of life you gain)
30. Everyone communicates a few connect: What the most effective people do differently	John Maxwell	February 2011 82.5 kg	Give people an action plan: ACT • Put a letter "A" beside those things you learned that you need to apply • Put a letter "C" beside those things you learned that you need to Change • Put a letter "I" besides those things you learned that you need to teach The way I like to measure greatness is …How many people can you make want better ? (Will Smith) Artist Walter Anderson observed " Our life improves only when we take chances and the first and most difficult risk we can take is to be honest with ourselves " Follow the Golden Rule: You need to treat people as you want to be treated
31. Strategies to succeed	Miguel Angel Cornejo	February 2011 82 kg	Leonardo : When fatigue and tiredness beat your body but your mind wants to continue, do not stop dreaming, convince yourself that life is full of stars. (page 88)

			Dreaming is an essential ingredient to achieve your life´s goals. To be able to create the first thing is to believe, to be able to dream with open eyes to see in our imagination what we wish. Faith is the cathalyst ingredient for creativity. For winners dreaming is of vital importance, they know that the dream is the origin of all achievement, big businesses are the result of a dream, of an obsession to crystalize wishes into reality In this life to achieve big goals it is necessary to be in love with your dreams
32. Make Today Count	John C. Maxwell	March 2011 81.5 kg	Discprepancies between values and practices create chaos in a person´s life. If you talk values but neglect to walk them, then you will continually undermine your integrity and credibility. You need to understand the Bible´s observation "Where your treasure is there your heart be also" and do like Benjamin Franklin, self-evaluate yourself at night versus the below daily dozen (or up to 20 core values) recommended by Maxwell, provided you started the day with this statement "What good will I do today ? " 1.Attitude 2.Priorities 3.Health 4.Family 5.Thinking 6.Commitment 7.Finances 8.Faith 9.Relationships 10.Generosity 11.Values 12.Growth
33. Long Walk to Freedom: The	Nelson Mandela	March 2011	A leader is a shepherd, stays behind the flock, letting the most

Autobiography of Nelson Mandela		80.5 kg	nimble going out ahead not realizing they are directed from behind A leader has to listen what every person in a discussion has to say before venturing his own opinion Neglecting one´s ancestors would bring ill-fortune and failure in life

As you can see I consistently lost 2 kg every month on average on a 12 month period. However it is worth noting the following:

1. I had to do a lot of reading beforehand

2. During summer time I relaxed the month after Spain won the World Cup which caused a pause in my progression during the month of August.

3. A magic water that I first drank in Johannesburg accelerated my progress in October 2010 when I lost 3 kg

4. The reading of Dale Carnegie´s How to Stop Worrying and Start Living relaxed me so much that I was able to lose 5 kg. You should be aware however that I bought this book in 2002 in a trip to the US. And yet I ignored it for about 8 years until October 2010. Here is the point: I am not an expert. I am human being like you who has learnt from his mistakes.

CHAPTER 3.Despite all the reading everything starts with Self-Talk

"Positive self-talk help you make changes in your life so you can move on by using the power of talking out loud to yourself"

Bill Wayne

"Evidence is conclusive that your self-talk has a direct bearing on your performance."

Zig Ziglar

"The Self-Talk that helps you to solve your problems is the same self-talk which will help you to reach your goals"

Shad Helmstetter

"By changing your self-talk you are changing your future and by changing your future you are changing your life "

Shad Helmstetter

3.1 The use of youtube.com as the World´s second largest search engine

Most people are unaware of the fact that already in August 2008, youtube.com overcame Yahoo as the World´s second largest search engine. ComScore's most U.S. search engine Rankings for August 2008 suggest that YouTube achieves a greater level of search traffic than Yahoo. If you were to consider YouTube's integrated search a regular search engine, you would have to hand Google the top two spots for search engine traffic. In combination, Google has about four times the search traffic of Yahoo and more than ten times the search traffic of Microsoft's MSN sites.

I only found out in 2010.

I then decided to search for my favorite authors in youtube.com. One of them is Shad Helmstetter. He is the author of the book "What to say when you talk to yourself". You can purchase it in the Internet as a used book for just 0.01 $.

The video from Shad Helmstetter which inspired me is this one

Dr. Shad Helmstetter - "The Story of Self-Talk"

http://www.youtube.com/watch?v=rvzfnm9uk-0

It is just a 7 minute video where he explains

1. How your brain work since you were born
2. The law of repetition
3. How he lost a lot of weight by self-talking and recording it and playing it while shaving

3.2 The use of self-recording to lose weight while reading Self-talk

I therefore said to myself. If as stated in the video Eastern European athletes could do it, I can do it as a Spanish world champion. And I started to self-record it myself every night saying "Tomorrow I will weight xxxx kg" I usually put a daily target i.e. I would lose 0.2 kg a day. As result I lost 13 kg between October and November 2010.

Warning to the reader: I am not a magician. I had read this book 3 times before over a period of 7 years. I had to re-read for the fourth time. I had to record it and open a tape called Self Talk for Weight Loss. I had to complement it with a tape called SW "Stop Worrying" (based on the book by Dale Carnegie: How to Stop Worrying and Start Living".

But the factual truth is that the final sentence of the above video from Shad

By changing your self-talk you are changing your future and by changing your future you are changing your life

proved to be 100% true in my case.

Whereas I would wholeheartedly recommend you to read the whole book from Shad Helmstetter, I would like to make it easier for you. This is the sentence which captivated me.

"You are responsible for lifting the fork, no one else is"

As a result I started to eat slower. I started to think before I did something I had not done in 44 years of my life.

3.3 The five steps of self-talk which brought my life back to health

When I read the statement from Shad that "We control with our minds most everything in our lives, including our HEALTH, our PERSONAL relationships, our careers and our futures" I went ahead and applied his 5 step program to my daily living.

Concepts relationship	Application	Result
1. Programming creates belief	**Programming** Medicines OK Check ups OK Driving OK Friends OK Work home OK Carmen we know the situation OK	**Belief** Health cannot be an issue as we wrote in the MOTB sell myself to myself commercial Sleeping well is a fact for 5 nights now (i.e. Wed night to Sat night inclusive) Health is quite all right as evidenced by jogging twice a day, several walks a day, supermarket visits and driving under rain even
2. Belief creates attitudes	**Belief** I can do everything myself as always I can handle the situations without maximizing the variables as we have learnt I can move on with the work front in the coming days	**Attitudes** There is no case for having fear when staying at home or walking If wake up in mid-nigh, drink hot drinks and take the medicine, no watches looked at Start with the plan of companies and then Mr Block but first companies well thought on
3. Attitudes creates feelings	**Attitudes** With a determine attitude all goes back to normal, or even better the euphoria will appear	**Feelings** Feel yourself euphoric you came back as TS said, enthusiasm makes things 1100% better
4. Feelings determine actions	**Feelings** Euphoria and enthusiasm feeling	**Actions** Non stopping i.e. if the day of flight I was in action from 11 to 22 hours; what stops me from being in action same number of hours?
5. Actions create results	**Actions** By being active the ultimate result is the confirmation of a much better life than before	**Results** With 20 kg less my life will be normal as before but much better in all respects and outcomes

As you can see I wrote 20 kg less. Overall I lost 28 kg. Dreams do come true.

3.4 How the self-talk was complemented with Stop Worrying the month afterwards

However although dreams do come true, fears appear always along the way. In order to build from the work I did in October 2010 while reading to Shad Helmstetter, I still had to make a major breakthrough in November 2010 through Dale Carnegie´s How to Stop Worrying and Start Living. In addition I put the acronym SW that Ronnie Kagan (http://au.linkedin.com/in/ronniekagan CEO of the Mentor Club) taught us at a leadership convention in Germany.

SW =Some won´t. Six will So what..
And transformed SW into
Stop worrying

How to Stop worrying and start living

By Dale Carnegie

Every day is a new life to a wise man

SALUTATION TO THE DAWN
Look to this day !
For it is life, the very life of life
In its brief course
Lie all the verities and realities of your existence
The bliss of growth
The glory of action
The splendor of beauty
For yesterday it is but a dream
And tomorrow is only a vision
But today well lived makes every yesterday a dream of happiness
And every tomorrow a vision of hope
Look well, therefore, to this day !
Such is the salutation to the dawn

Kalidasa

Here is the full index of the book which I encourage you to buy in English or any language around the world. I have seen it in German and Spanish too.

Index

PART I   FUNDAMENTAL FACTS YOU SHOULD KNOW ABOUT WORRY

PART II   BASIC TECHNIQUES IN ANALYZING WORRY

PART III   HOW TO BREAK THE WORRY HABIT BEFORE IT BREAKS YOU

PART IV   SEVEN WAYS TO CULTIVATE A MENTAL ATTITUDE THAT WILL BRING YOU PEACE AND HAPPINESS

PART V   THE PERFECT WAY TO CONQUER WORRY

PART VI   HOW TO KEEP WORRYING ABOUT CRITICISM

PART VII   HOW TO KEEP WORRYING ABOUT CRITICISM

PART VIII   HOW I CONQUERED WORRY

Final warning: If you think for a moment that this is a book for psychologists you are dead wrong. As a veteran of the Corporate World I would tell you that this book is a must read for any CEO, CFO, CIO, SVP etc…of any company. Therefore I would urge you to purchase it to put your life and your business in order.

CHAPTER 4.Water the ultimate cure

"Water is the driving force of all nature"

Da Vinci

"Water absorbs negativity"

John Gray

4.1 The discovery Steve Meyerowitz in 2004

In 2004 I was conducting a professional assignment in Italy. The assignment took long i.e. non stopping from April to November 2004. This means that effectively I was flying in and out of Italy during spring, summer and autumn. I was most of the time in the Ligurian region

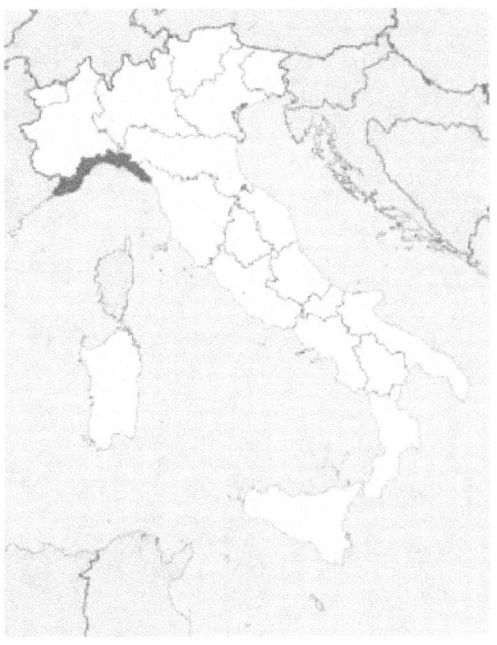

Liguria borders France to the west, Piedmont to the north, and Emilia-Romagna and Tuscany to the east. It lies on the Ligurian Sea. The narrow strip of land is bordered by the sea, the Alps and the Apennines mountains. Some mountains rise above 2000 m; the watershed line runs at an average altitude of about 1000 m.

The winding arched extension goes from Ventimiglia to La Spezia and is one of the smallest regions in Italy. Liguria is just 5,422 square kilometres, or 1.18% of all of Italy. Of this, 3524.08 kilometres are mountainous (65% of the total) and 891.95 square kilometres are hills (35% of the total). Liguria's Natural Reserves cover 12% of the entire region, or 60,000 hectares of land. They are made up of one National Reserve, six large parks, two smaller parks and three nature reserves.

The continental shelf is very narrow, and so steep it descends almost immediately to considerable marine depths along its 315-km coastline. Except for thePortovenere and Portofino promontories, it is generally not very jagged, and is often high. At the mouths of the biggest watercourses there are small beaches, but there are no deep bays and natural harbours except for those of Genoa and La Spezia.

The ring of hills lying immediately beyond the coast together with the sea account for a mild climate year-round. Average winter temperatures are 7 to 10 °C (45 to 50 °F) and summer temperatures of 23 to 24 °C (73 to 75 °F), which make for a pleasant stay even in the dead of winter. Rainfall can be abundant at times, as mountains very close to the coast create an orographic effect. Genoa and La Spezia can see up to 2,000 mm (79 in) of rain in a year; other areas instead show the normal Mediterranean rainfall of 500 to 800 mm (20 to 31 in) annually.

I went there with a weight of approximately 98 kg and within a few months I put 12 kg more to 112 kg. As you can imagine I struggled during summer time because despite the aforementioned average temperatures the truth of the matter is that in summer is actually much hotter and with plenty of humidity.

It was on a weekend trip to Holland when I encountered the below book

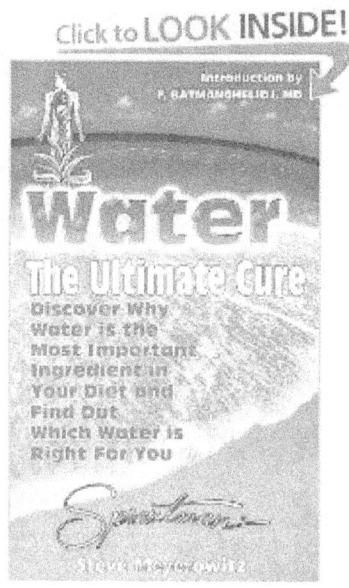

by Steve Meyerowitz **http://www.linkedin.com/pub/steve-meyerowitz/12/386/151**

Despite being a persistent book reader the only reason I bought the book was …the inspiration from the Providence. I guess it was the front page and the pictures of the beaches which reminded me of the need to swim in the Italian sea during my assignment. I wholeheartedly recommend you the book. It inspired me a lot with the following advices from Steve Meyerowitz

4.1.1 The 10 Commandments of Good Hydration according to Steve Meyerowitz

1. Drink ½ ounce daily for every pound you weigh. A 150lb person drinks 75 ounces, or approximately 2.5 quarts. One glass every hour is a good rule of thumb.

2. Avoid diuretic beverages that flush water out of your body, such as caffeinated coffee, tea, soda, pop, alcohol or beer.

3. Drink more water, and fresh juices to maintain hydration during illness and upon recovery. Illness robs your body of water.

4. Start your day with ½ to 1 quart of water to flush your digestive tract and rehydrate your system from the overnight fast.

5. Drink water at regular intervals throughout the day. Don´t wait until you are thirsty. Thirst indicates an already present deficiency.

6. Get in the habit of carrying a water bottle with you or keep one in the car or on your desk. Convenience helps. Stuff it in your shoulder bag or waist pack bottle pocket. Hiking suppliers have a nice selection of water-bearing belt packs and accessories.

7. Make a habit of drinking water. According to a survey, the reason most people don´t drink as much as they know they ought to, is lack of time or being too busy. Decide to drink water before every meal. Set objectives for yourself such as drinking before you leave the house, and first thing upon your return or before you start work. Take water breaks instead of coffee breaks. Fill a size glass you can finish or gauge yourself by the number of water bottles you drink during the day.

8. Increase your drinking when you increase your mental activity level; your stress level; your exercise level.

9. Drink the purest water available.

10. Perspire. Exercise to the point of perspiration or enjoy a steam bath. Sweat cleans the lymphatic system and bloodstream. It is one of the best detoxification avenues available to us. Do sweat and do drink plenty of water afterwards to replace the loss of fluids. Drink more in hot weather.

4.1.2 How Much to Drink? According to Steve Meyerowitz

The average adult should drink from 2-3 ½ quarts (liters) of high quality, pure water daily.

One possible way to break it up is

1. Drink half a liter in the morning before breakfast. This is great flush of your intestines and helps prepare the stomach for food and avoids constipation.

2. Drink half a liter 3 hours after breakfast

3. Take another half liter 20 minutes before lunch.

4. Drink half a liter 3 hours after lunch

5. Take another half liter 20 minutes before dinner

Despite taking those notes from Steve´s book I still failed to lose weight. In retrospect the reason has to do with something that I have read in Zig Ziglar´s Secrets of closing the sale: We speak to ourselves some 4.800 words every 24 hours. And yet 3.200 are about ourselves in a negative way. This makes us not to pay attention to key details. In my case I forgot all what Steve says with regards the coffee or clean diet. However I did memorize 3 things i.e.

1. To carry water with me at all times
2. To think that if I am thirsty I mean I am dehydrated
3. To know that I have to drink 3 litres of water a day

Out of ignorance I also missed what Steve says above i.e. drink the purest possible water. I went on and on to buy stilled water in Italy but until 2010 I did not understand what pure water was.

Therefore I kept myself content with research via the following website.

4.2   Watercure.com by Dr. Fereydoon Batmanghelidj

Watercure.com belongs to **Fereydoon Batmanghelidj, M.D.**, an internationally renowned researcher, author and advocate of the natural healing power of water, was born in Iran in 1931. He attended Fettes College in Scotland and was a graduate of St. Mary's Hospital Medical School of London University, where he studied under Sir Alexander Fleming, who shared the Nobel Prize for the discovery of penicillin.

Dr. Batmanghelidj practiced medicine in the United Kingdom before returning to Iran where he played a key role in the development of hospitals and medical centers. He also helped establish sport projects for youth in Iran, including The Ice Palace in Tehran, the first ice skating and sports complex in the Middle East.

I wholeheartedly recommend you to read the website, and read his books as well as the podcasts from America´s top leadership guru Tonny Robbins. Here are some of the tips from Dr Batmanghelidj

1. You're not sick; you're thirsty. Don't treat thirst with medication."

2. Our life, our planet. Over 70% of the earth's surface is water. However, most of it—98%--is salt water. Only 2% of the earth's H20 is fresh water that we can

44

drink, and of this, almost all is trapped in frozen glaciers.

3. You are not just what you eat; you are what you drink. This is why water is so important to your health.

4. Water is the basis of all life and that includes your body. Your muscles that move your body are 75% water; your blood that transport nutrients is 82% water; your lungs that provide your oxygen are 90% water; your brain that is the control center of your body is 76% water; even your bones are 25% water.

5. Our health is truly dependent on the quality and quantity of the water we drink.

6. If you are committed to a healthy lifestyle, make drinking enough natural water a habit in your life. It won't take long for you to feel the benefit. It is a free investment for your long-term health.

Again, although the advices are invaluable, I missed key things. I stuck to Donald Trump´s principle of You are what you eat (in his book How to Get Rich). But I got it wrong. It is what you drink. I drank plenty of Italian water San Benedetto which pleased my Italian friend Daniele Lorenzini. But yet I kept on putting weight to insurmountable levels.

4.3 The pursuit of a dream took me to a discovery Johannesburg in July 2011

9th July 2010. I land in Johannesburg, South Africa. Within 45 minutes of landing I am one of Spain´s more satisfied men. André Paris http://za.linkedin.com/pub/andre-paris/22/ab7/278 owner of www.chezparis.co.za takes me directly from the airport to FIFA ticketing point. Without queuing up, I get my prepaid tickets from FIFA. I had prepaid them in January 2010. Something inside me told me that Spain would play the final in Johannesburg. It was 11 am and I had plenty of time to enjoy this beautiful house in Johannesburg

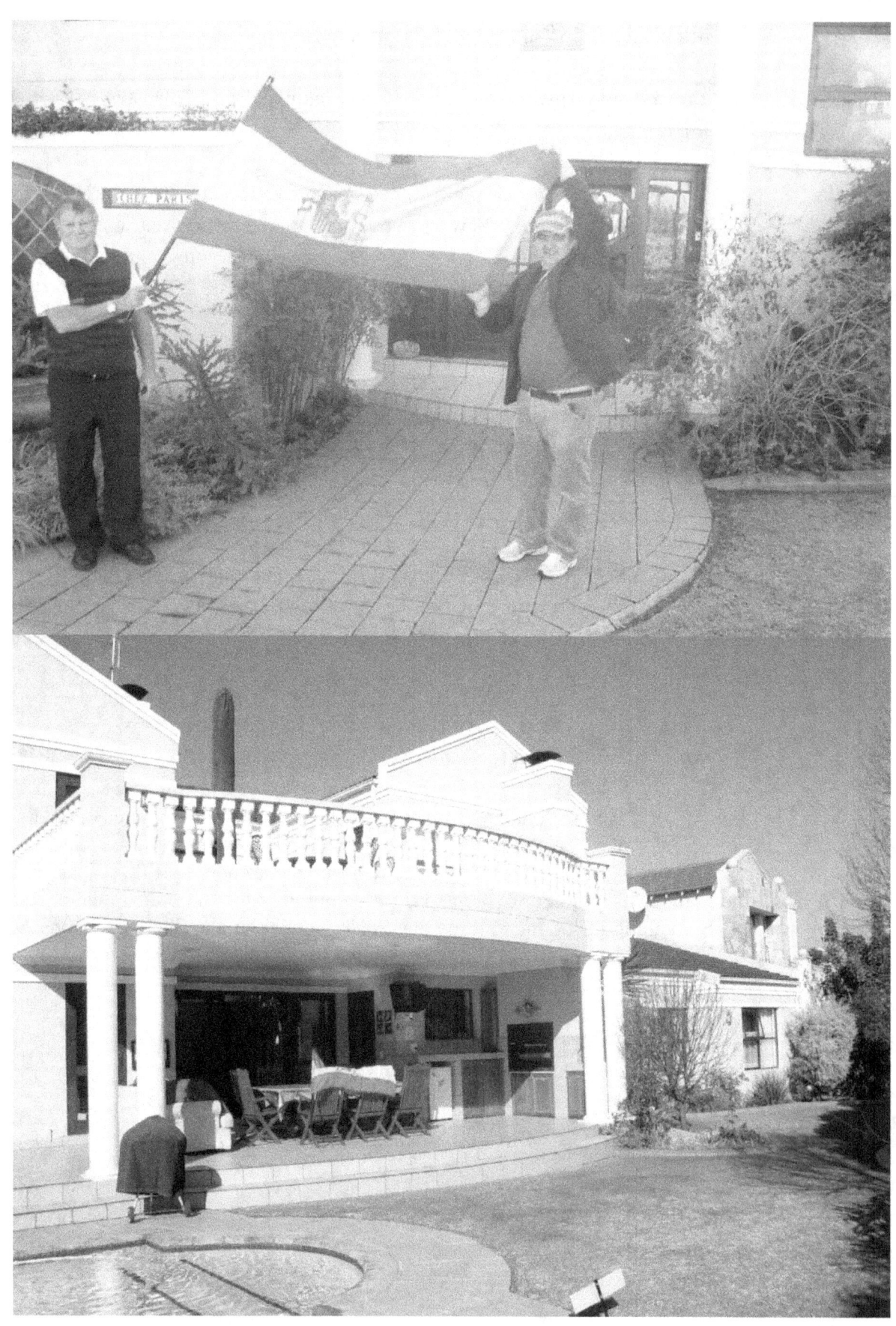

André checked me in and introduced me to his wonderful wife Lizette who gave me the best possible room in the house including a personal terrace as you can see above.

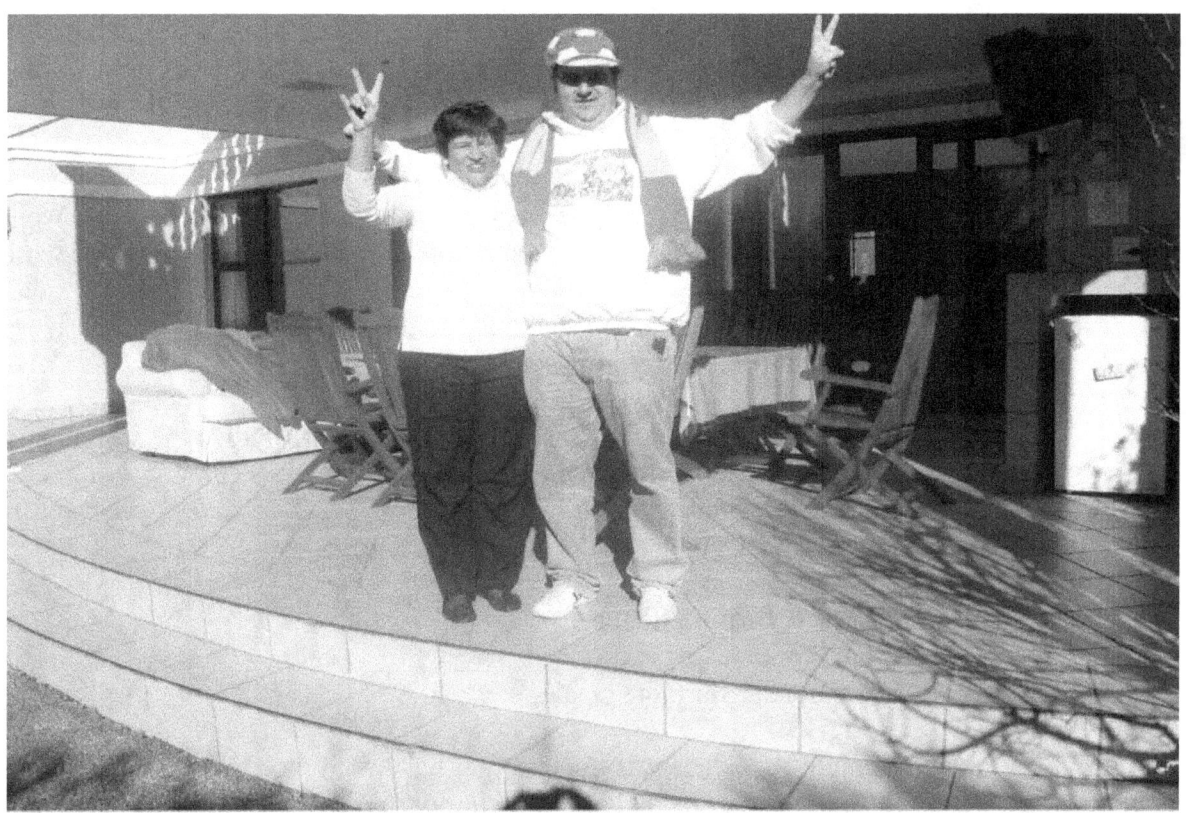

They gently gave me time to get changed, have a shower, a coffee and drive to the nearest restaurant for lunch. After a first class drop-off and pick-up to return to the house for a Spanish siesta (nap) André said these words in very shy terms "This is the best water in the world…and he served me the water in a jug from the below espring purifier"

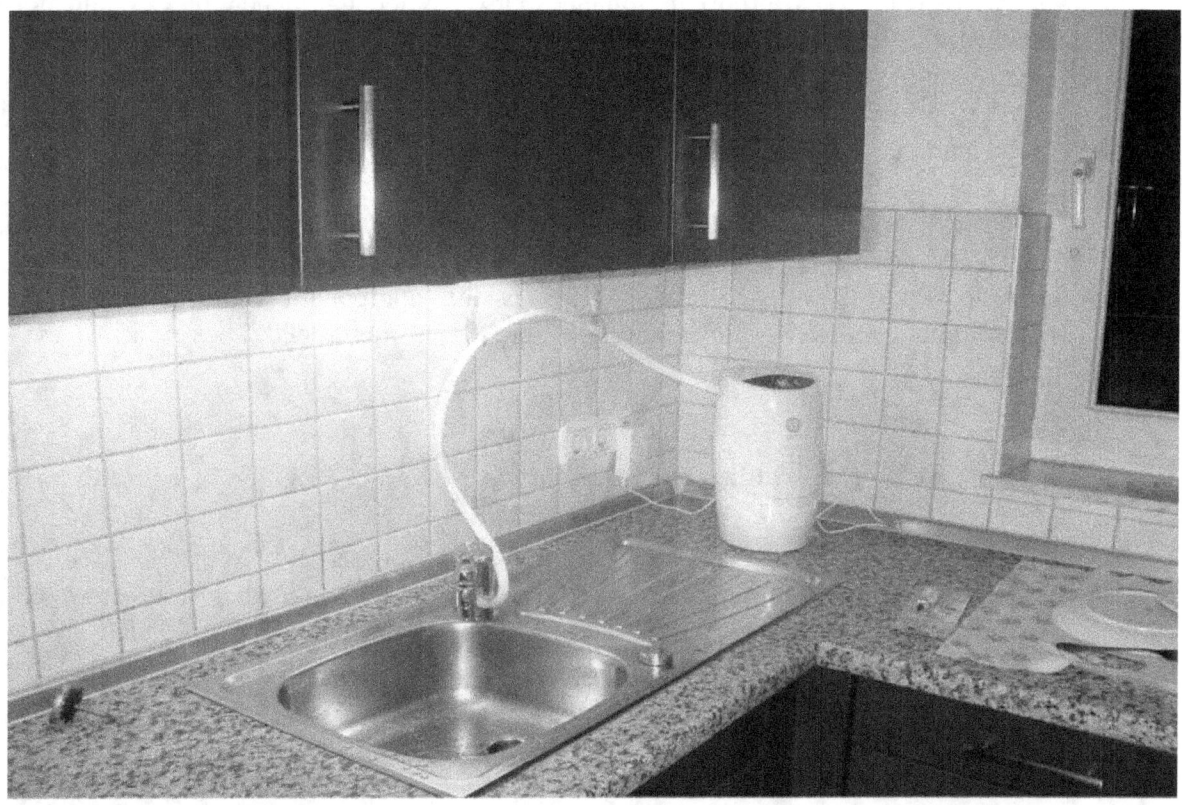

When I was drinking the water I had no idea that this was espring.com (which self-defines itself as the best source of water at home). I simply took the water, kept on drinking and went to sleep.

After 2-3 hours I woke up. I had the luxury of a enjoying a stay in a suite which was much better than any suite at the many 4 star hotels I have been to around the world.

I was feeling great with the outstanding quality of the water. Yet I was not understanding that much. My ignorance prevailed.

I went to the kitchen of the house (the above is my kitchen) studied the system a little bit and became impressed with the microchip and ultraviolet technology of the espring purifier. But still I did not relate to it. I open a cupboard to have a glass and I saw a bunch of vitamins in the cupboard.

The brand name was familiar to me.

Nutrilite. See chapter 5 for more details.

Because that night the house was going to get busy with more World Cup visitors I did not speak to André and Lizette about it. I simply said that the water was outstanding. I still could not relate espring to Nutrilite. Besides it was a World Cup final weekend and I had no time for these things. In addition the last 2 nights (after the victorious game at Soccer City where Spain became World Champions) were spent at another house nearby the Paris family.

But on Tuesday 13th July (who said that is bad date) 2010, Lizette Paris gently drove me to Oliver Tambo´s airport in Johannesburg. When I told her that I could not relate Nutrilite to espring, and that I could even less expect "that thing to be in Africa" she drove me via the highway to see the South African headquarters of American Way (www.amway.com). She explained that this business existed in South Africa, Bostwana and Nambia.

In conclusion I was such an ignorant that despite knowing Nutrilite (but not taking a single vitamin since 2007) I had to fly all the way down to Johannesburg to learn of the world´s purest water espring. This is the component I was missing from the recommendations of Steve and Dr Fereydoon mentioned above: drink the purest possible water.

4.4 The effect of drinking the World´s purest water: 8 kg loss in 2 months

As stated before in chapter 3 I lost some 8 kg in October and November 2010. Whereas everything was important, the critical ingredient was indeed the purest water in the world. This time I made no mistake. I persistently drank 3 litres of water. To do that I have 8 bottles of 1.5 litres permanently available in my kitchen. I take them with me everywhere. That why I ensure that I always drink 3 litres of waters per day. Here the evidence in my kitchen.

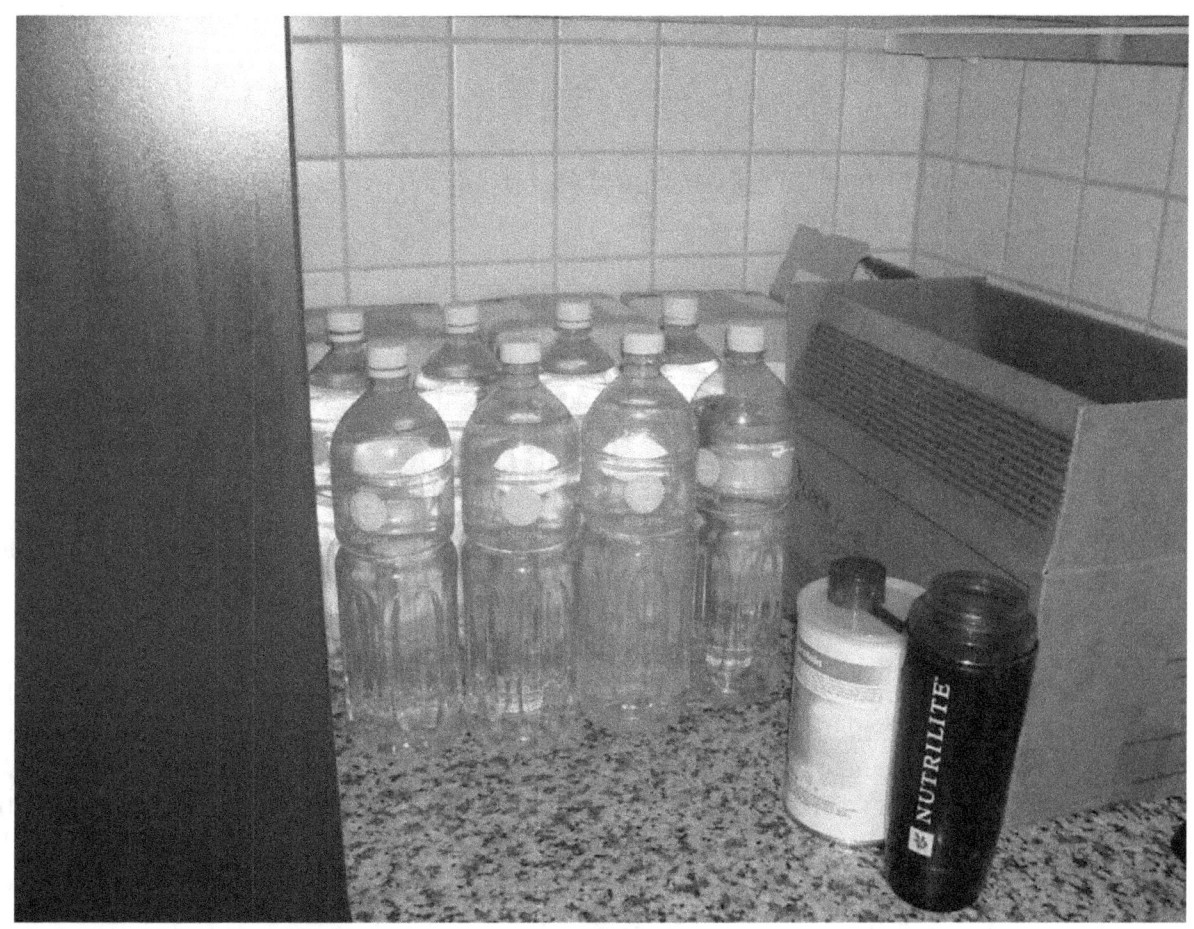

4.4.1 Yotube.com videos which evidence what pure water is versus any other tap of water

Once again the habit of using youtube.com as the World´s second largest search engine proves critical to understand what pure water is.

Here a list of must see videos:

eSpring Water Filter/Filtration System Best Benchtop/Undersink Home Purifer/Purifying

Uploaded by intafitness on Apr 3, 2010

http://www.youtube.com/watch?v=AqZ8rzjfHZw

eSpring - the world's best source of water

Uploaded by insider201283 on Nov 24, 2006

http://www.youtube.com/watch?v=JhdOexEHfgM

eSpring® - The Best Water Purifier – Demo

Uploaded by soumen81 on Apr 23, 2008

Perfect Water

This latest video will leave you high and dry if you are still skeptic. It basically tells you to pay attention. Whether you are drinking bottled water or tap water you are still drinking a product of a certain technology. It can be the technology used by a company or the technology used by municipal authorities.

None of them has the microchip and ultraviolet technology which espring.com offers in their website.

You have to realize that the parent company of espring, the holding Alticor and the flagship Amway do in excess of 9 billion dollars of sales every year. And as I mentioned earlier they go as far down as to South Africa. The high –tech capabilities of this conglomerate of enterprises is far superior to any other multinational in the world. Whatever they market is exclusive, and they come up with the best value added offer to the consumer.

4.4.2 Public information available at the World´s purest water website

The website espring.com is broken down into the following sections:

- Home
- Water Wellness
- Why espring
- Products
- Research Center
- Opportunity
- Customer Service

For each section I wholeheartedly recommend you to research and read every single section. Thus for instance in the section Why espring the break-down is as follows:

The Best Source

True Innovation

UV Light

Carbon Filter

Monitor

Performance Claims

The best source section contains invaluable information such as:

Why choose an eSpring™ Water Purifier? The answer is simple: because the eSpring Water Purifier is *the world's best source of water*. You can be confident that the water your family drinks is as clean as it can possibly be, and that it has met the highest standards for clean water quality.

- The eSpring Water Purifier destroys more than 99.99% of waterbourne, disease-causing bacteria and viruses in drinking water
- Water from the eSpring Water Purifier is safer than tap water
- It dramatically improves the taste, odour and clarity of water
- Other systems treat drinking water, eSpring purifies it

There are many reasons to choose an eSpring Water Purifier.

In addition to the benefits listed above, the eSpring Water Purifier also:
- reduces potential carcinogens that can be found in drinking water
- is more convenient than bottled water
- has a high flow rate to fill your glass or container quickly
- treats drinking/cooking water for a family of 6 for up to one year
- improves the taste of beverages made with filtered water
- is convenient and easy to operate
- has a smart, sleek, space-saving design
- has convenient and easy replacements
- is less costly than bottled water
- has been certified to reduce potential health effect contaminants than any other carbon based system.
- effectively reduces chlorine
- effectively reduces lead in drinking water
- effectively reduces mercury in drinking water
- effectively reduces waterbourne parasites
- effectively reduces radon and radon decay products in drinking water
- does not remove beneficial minerals, such as calcium, magnesium, and fluoride
- uses exclusive patented technology
- is designed, assembled and manufactured in the USA
- comes with a satisfaction guaranteed or your money back

No other Water Purifier compares to the eSpring Water Purifier.

The eSpring Water Purifier is truly the first of its kind in many respects:
- The **first** company to develop in-home system's that combine a patented carbon-block filter with ultraviolet light and an electronic monitoring system
- the **only** system verified to effectively remove lead, THMs and more than 140 contaminants
- the **first** company in the world to have a carbon/UV system that meets NSF International Standards 42, 53 and 55 - three internationally recognized water quality standards
- certified by NSF International for the reduction of **more contaminants than any other UV carbon based system**
- the **first** system to use wireless inductive coupling technology to increase safety and reliability

The question for you is: Do you think that a conglomerate of that prestige would make those statements in their website if they were untrue ?

I will answer for you: No they would not

I will again remind you my experience: Despite drinking other waters and keeping in mind what I learnt from Steve and Fereydoon I still missed what pure water means. I hope you are smarter than me.

CHAPTER 5. Vitamin supplements

"Balance energy throughout the day with smaller more frequent meals and water"

Twitter.com/Nutrilitehealth

The combination of vitamins such as daily multivitamin supplements, omega 3 and Vitamin B proved very positive for my health.

5.1 Daily multivitamin supplement

Here is the standard definition from Wikipedia:

5.1.1 What is a multivitamin ?

A multivitamin is a preparation intended to supplement a human diet with vitamins, dietary minerals, and other nutritional elements. Such preparations are available in the form of tablets, capsules, pastilles, powders, liquids, and injectable formulations. Other than injectable formulations, which are only available and administered under medical supervision, multivitamins are recognized by the Codex Alimentarius Commission (the United Nations' authority on food standards) as a category of food. Multivitamin supplements are commonly provided in combination with dietary minerals. A multivitamin/mineral supplement is defined in the United States as a supplement containing 3 or more vitamins and minerals that does not include herbs, hormones, or drugs, where each vitamin and mineral is included at a dose below the tolerable upper level, as determined by the Food and Drug Board, and does not present a risk of adverse health effects. The terms multivitamin and multimineral are often used interchangeably. There is no scientific definition for either.

5.1.2 Which products and components form multivitamins?

Many multivitamins are formulated or labeled to differentiate consumer sectors, such as prenatal, children, mature or 50+, men's, women's, diabetic, or stress. Consumer multivitamin formulas are available as tablets, capsules, bulk powder, or liquid. Most multivitamins are intended to be taken once or twice per day, although some formulations are designed for consumption 3–7 or more times per day.

Compositional variation amongst brands and lines allows substantial consumer choices. Modern multivitamin products roughly classify into RDA (recommended dietary allowance) centric multivitamins with or without iron, RDA centric multivitamin/multimineral formulas with or without iron, higher potency formulas with mostly above RDA components with or without iron, and more specialized formulas by condition, such as for diabetics or by less common components, such as diversified antioxidants, herbal extracts, or premium vitamin and mineral forms. Legally, the United States Food and Drug Administration allows a multivitamin to be called "high potency" if at least two-thirds of its nutrients have at least 100 percent of the DV. In practice, "high potency" usually means substantially increased vitamins C and B, with some other enhanced vitamin and mineral levels, though some minerals may still be much less than DV.

Some components are typically much lower than RDA amounts, often for cost reasons. For example, biotin, usually the most expensive vitamin component, at over $4000 per active pound, is typically added in at only 5%-30% of RDA in many one per day formulations. Biotin is required to be present at 100% of the value of the B-vitamins for them to be absorbed by the body. Any B-vitamins that cannot be absorbed due to a lack of biotin are eliminated by the body. Likewise, boron and magnesium are considered essential for the bioavailability and absorption of Vitamin D and calcium. Sometimes low content composition is for population subgroups, where the RDA would be inappropriate. Iron is needed in larger amounts by menstruating women, but some percentage of HFE variant gene bearing males are at risk for hemochromatosis. Normal dietary intakes also vary by population, indicating different levels of supplementation.

Basic commercial multivitamin supplement products often contain the following ingredients:

- vitamin C, B_1, B_2, B_3, B_6, folic acid (B_9), B_{12}, B_5 (pantothenate),

- H (biotin), A, E, D_3, K_1, potassium iodide, cupric (sulfate anhydrous, picolinate, sulfate monohydrate, trioxide)

- selenomethionine, borate(s), zinc, calcium, magnesium, chromium, manganese, molybdenum, betacarotene, and iron.

- Other formulas may include additional ingredients such as other carotenes (*e.g.* lutein, lycopene), higher than RDA amounts of B, C or E vitamins including gamma-tocopherol, "near" B vitamins (inositol, choline, PABA), trimethylglycine (anhydrous betaine), betaine hydrochloride, vitamin K_2 as menaquinone-7, lecithin, citrus bioflavinoids or nutrient forms variously described as more easily absorbed.

5.1.3 Health-benefits associated to multivitamins

In 2002, a paper by Robert H. Fletcher and Kathleen M. Fairfield from the Harvard School of Medicine, in the Journal of the American Medical Association stated that "it appears prudent for all adults to take vitamin supplements." In this article, which examined the clinical applications of vitamins for the prevention of chronic diseases in adults examined English-language articles about vitamins in relation to chronic diseases published between 1966 and 2002, and concluded that inadequate intake of several vitamins has been linked to the development of diseases including coronary heart disease, cancer, and osteoporosis.

Similarly, the April 9, 1998 issue of the New England Journal of Medicine featured an editorial entitled "Eat Right and Take a Multivitamin" that was based on studies that showed health benefits resulting from the consumption of supplemental folate to prevent birth defects and possibly decrease the incidence of cardiovascular disease.

A 2007 UC Berkeley School of Public Health study in collaboration with Shaklee Corporation determined that long-term vitamin and mineral supplement users showed markedly better health than people who took no supplements. "After adjustment for age, gender, income, education and body mass index, greater degree of supplement use was associated with more favorable concentrations of serum homocysteine, C-reactive protein, high-density lipoprotein cholesterol, and triglycerides, as well as lower risk of prevalent elevated blood pressure and diabetes."

There is a new gravitation in the United States towards the Mediterranean diet. This diet is based on the Mediterranean Diet Pyramid, created by Walter Willett in 1995. In 2008, the Harvard School of Public Health updated Willett's pyramid in a Nutrition Source article called "Food Pyramids: What Should You Really Eat?". Included in this new pyramid, and the original pyramid, is a daily multivitamin. The Harvard article states that "A daily multivitamin, multi-mineral supplement offers a kind of nutritional backup, especially when it includes some extra vitamin D. While a multivitamin can't in any way replace healthy eating, or make up for unhealthy eating, it can fill in the nutrient holes that may sometimes affect even the most careful eaters."[21]

A 2009 study published in *The American Journal of Clinical Nutrition* reports that multivitamin use is associated with longer telomere length in women. Longer telomeres have recently been associated with longer life, and therefore multivitamins could have an anti-aging effect. However, this is the first study on this topic, so more studies must be done to confirm this effect.

In response to a 2009 study stating the uselessness of multivitamins, the Linus Pauling Institute published an article refuting the study's legitimacy and claims. According to the Linus Pauling Institute, the 2009 study was an observational study, not a randomized controlled trial. "Every epidemiologist will tell you that observational studies cannot establish cause-and-effect relationships; they only can observe associations." Additionally, 41.5 percent of the female participants took multivitamins and were overall healthier in all their habits . This makes it difficult to separate their healthy habits from their multivitamin use. Perhaps they used multivitamins because they already had healthy habits and were therefore healthier overall. The Linus Pauling article concludes with this statement: "Even Dr. JoAnn Manson, a principal investigator of the Women's Health Initiative and co-author of the study, acknowledges that 'the research doesn't mean multivitamins are useless. Multivitamins may still be useful as a form of [health] insurance for people with poor eating habits.' And let's not fool ourselves, that's the large majority of the people in this country!"

Bruce Ames, professor of Biochemistry and Molecular Biology at the University of California, Berkeley, and a senior scientist at Children's Hospital Oakland Research Institute (CHORI), suggests that "to maximize human health and lifespan, scientists must abandon outdated models of micronutrients" and that "a metabolic tune-up through an improved supply of micronutrients is likely to have great health benefits

5.1.4 October 2010: The multivitamin that I had stopped taking in 2007

In October 2010 I started taking a multivitamin called Double X. I had stopped taking this vitamin in 2007 out of an illness which kept me in Spain for several months. It was a crucial mistake because Double X has had proven success for decades.

In 1934, Carl Rehnborg originated the concept of including whole plant concentrates in his formula for the first multivitamin/multimineral product sold in North America. In 1948, NUTRILITE introduced its premier product, called DOUBLE X. The formulation for DOUBLE X is based on Carl Rehnborg's early nutritional research, and still includes alfalfa, parsley, and other plant materials he recognized as being nutritionally beneficial.

DOUBLE X is Nutrilite´s flagship product and its formula is updated regularly, based on the nutritional research being done by NUTRILITE scientists around the world.

DOUBLE X is designed around a simple nutritional principle: To provide an essential nutritional foundation for people who understand the many benefits provided by vitamins, minerals, and plant concentrates (phytonutrients). The key product benefits are

- People depend on DOUBLE X because of its sound nutritional basis:
- DOUBLE X is power-packed with vitamins, minerals, and plant concentrates, supporting your active and healthy lifestyle.
- DOUBLE X has phytonutrients with antioxidant protection, targeting key groups of cell-damaging free radicals.

In Japan, this product is named NUTRILITE TRIPLE X.

The results on my health were positive almost instantaneously. I had much more energy to jog daily. Right now I wake up at 5 am. At 6 am I drive to the municipal pool. I take Double X with a Protein Bar and an Isotonic drink. That keeps me going for 2 hours till breakfast time at 8 am. Since the moment I started with Double X to March 2010 I lost almost 20 kg.

The reasons behind my success are explained in this video. You can see athletes like Asafa Powell or Doctors like Duke Johnson talking about the benefits of Double X

Nutrilite - Double-X

http://www.youtube.com/watch?v=tWVEpbtwITQ

Uploaded by zilim on Aug 1, 2007

In addition the below video

NUTRILITE® DOUBLE X® Vitamin/Mineral/Phytonutrient
http://www.youtube.com/watch?v=ptXYeZQ5kLg

Uploaded by prohomebasedbusiness on Feb 12, 2010
http://glapena.qhealthbeauty.com/

gives a full explanation as to why the Double X is the perfect multivitamin complement for a balance diet

In my case I will put it very simple to you: Double X gives me enough vitamins which makes me to avoid eating things that I should not eat.

5.2 Omega 3

Here is the standard definition from Wikipedia:

5.2.1 What is an Omega 3 vitamin?

Fish oil is oil derived from the tissues of oily fish. Fish oils contain the omega-3 fatty acids eicosapentaenoic acid (EPA), and docosahexaenoic acid (DHA), precursors of certain eicosanoids that are known to reduce inflammation throughout the body, and are thought to have many health benefits.

Fish do not actually produce omega-3 fatty acids, but instead accumulate them by consuming either microalgae or prey fish that have accumulated omega-3 fatty acids, together high quantity of antioxidants as iodide and selenium, from microalgae, where these antioxidants are able to protect the fragile polyunsaturated lipids from peroxidation . Fatty predatory fish like sharks, sword fish, tilefish, and albacore tuna may be high in omega-3 fatty acids, but due to their position at the top of the food chain, these species can also accumulate toxic substances (see biomagnification). For this reason, the U.S. Food and Drug Administration recommends limiting consumption of certain (predatory) fish species (e.g. albacore tuna, shark, king mackerel, tilefish and swordfish) due to high levels of toxic contaminants such as mercury, dioxin, PCBs and chlordane. Fish oil is used as a component in aquaculture feed. More than 50 percent of the world's fish oil used in aquaculture feed is fed to farmed salmon.

The omega-3 fatty acids in fish oil are thought to be beneficial in treating hypertriglyceridemia, and possibly beneficial in preventing heart disease. Fish oil and omega-3 fatty acids have been studied in a wide variety of other conditions, such as clinical depression, anxiety, cancer, and macular degeneration, although benefit in these conditions remains to be proven.

5.2.2 What are the health benefits associated to Omega 3 vitamin?

5.2.2.1 Cancer

Several studies report possible anti-cancer effects of $n-3$ fatty acids found in fish oil (particularly breast, colon and prostate cancer). Omega-3 fatty acids reduced prostate cancer growth, slowed histopathological progression, and increased survival in genetically engineered mice. Among n-3 fatty acids (omega-3), neither long-chain nor short-chain forms were consistently associated with reduced breast cancer risk. High levels of docosahexaenoic acid, however, the most abundant n-3 polyunsaturated fatty acid (omega-3) in erythrocyte membranes, were associated with a reduced risk of breast cancer. A recent study of 35,000 middle-aged women found that the women who took fish oil supplements had a 32% lower risk of breast cancer, although the authors stress the result is preliminary and falls short of establishing a causal relationship.

5.2.2.2 Cardiovascular

A 2008 meta-study by the *Canadian Medical Association Journal* found fish oil supplementation did not demonstrate any preventative benefit to cardiac patients with ventricular arrhythmias.

The American Heart Association recommends the consumption of 1g of fish oil daily, preferably by eating fish, for patients with coronary heart disease although pregnant and nursing women are advised to avoiding eating fish with high potential for mercury contaminants including mackerel, shark, or swordfish. Note that optimal dosage relates to body weight.

The US National Institutes of Health lists three conditions for which fish oil and other omega-3 sources are most highly recommended: hypertriglyceridemia, secondary cardiovascular disease prevention and high blood pressure. It then lists 27 other conditions for which there is less evidence. It also lists possible safety concerns: "Intake of 3 grams per day or greater of omega-3 fatty acids may increase the risk of bleeding, although there is little evidence of significant bleeding risk at lower doses. Very large intakes of fish oil/omega-3 fatty acids may increase the risk of hemorrhagic (bleeding) stroke.

There is also some evidence that fish oil may have a beneficial effect on some forms of cardiac dysrhythmia.

5.2.2.3 Mental Health

Studies published in 2004 and 2009 have suggested that the *n-3* EPA may reduce the risk of depression and suicide. One study compared blood samples of 100 suicide-attempt patients and to those of controls and found that levels ofEicosapentaenoic acid were significantly lower in the washed red blood cells of the suicide-attempt patients. A small American trial in 2009 suggested that E-EPA, as monotherapy, might treat major depressive disorder but failed to achieve statistical significance.

Studies were conducted on prisoners in England where the inmates were fed seafood which contains omega-3 fatty acids. The higher consumption of these fatty acids corresponded with a drop in the assault rates. Another Finnish study found that prisoners who were convicted of violence had lower levels of omega–3 fatty acids than prisoners convicted of nonviolent offenses. It was suggested that these kinds of fatty acids are responsible for the neuronal growth of the frontal cortex of the brain which, it is further alleged, is the seat of personal behavior.

A study from the Orygen Research Centre in Melbourne suggests that omega-3 fatty acids could also help delay or prevent the onset of schizophrenia. The researchers enlisted 81 'high risk' young people aged 13 to 24 who had previously suffered brief hallucinations or delusions and gave half of them capsules of fish oil while the other half received placebo. One year on, only three percent of those on fish oil had developed schizophrenia compared to 28 percent from those on placebo. A study conducted at Sheffield University in England reported positive results with fish oil on patients suffering from schizophrenia. Participants of the study had previously taken anti-psychotic prescription drugs that were no longer effective. After taking fish oil supplements, participants in the study experienced progress compared to others who were given a placebo.

The largest controlled study to date found no cognitive benefit after two years in the elderly.

5.2.2.4 Alzheimer´s disease

According to a study from Louisiana State University in September 2005, Docosahexaenoic acid, an omega-3 fatty acid often found in fish oil, may help protect the brain from cognitive problems associated with Alzheimer's disease.

5.2.2.5 Lupus

In a Northern Ireland study, lupus disease activity, especially in the skin and joints, was significantly reduced in patients who received fish oil supplements at both 12-week and 24-week follow-up periods versus patients who received placebo. There were also changes in the blood platelets of the patients who took the fish oil supplements, with an increase in proteins that are considered anti-inflammatory and a decrease in proteins that promote inflammation; these changes were not evident in the group that took placebo. The fish oil group showed an increase in FMD, which the researchers took as a sign that the omega-3 oils were helping the cells in the blood vessel walls to remain healthy.

5.2.2.6 Parkinson disease

A study examining whether omega-3 exerts neuroprotective action in Parkinson's disease found that it did exhibit a protective effect in mice. The scientists exposed mice to either a control or a high omega-3 diet from two to twelve months of age and then treated them with a neurotoxin commonly used as an experimental model for Parkinson's. The scientists found that high doses of omega-3 given to the experimental group prevented the neurotoxin-induced decrease of dopamine that ordinarily occurs. Since Parkinson's is a disease caused by disruption of the dopamine system, this protective effect exhibited could show promise for future research in the prevention of Parkinson's disease.

5.2.2.7 Depression

Evidence regarding the efficacy of fish oil supplements as a treatment for depression is inconclusive. Whereas several methodologically rigorous studies have reported statistically significant positive effects in the treatment of depressed patients, other studies have found effects to be insignificant.

An August 2003 double-blind placebo-controlled study published in the journal *European Neuropsychopharmacology* found that among 28 patients with major depressive disorder, "patients in the omega-3 PUFA group had a significantly decreased score on the 21-item Hamilton Rating Scale for Depression than those in the placebo group. Another study in the *American Journal of Psychiatry* reported that the addition of fish oil supplements to regular maintenance anti-depression therapy conferred "highly significant" benefits by the third week of the trial.

In contrast, a 2005 randomized double-blind placebo-controlled study conducted under the auspices of the New Zealand Institute for Crop & Food Research found "no evidence that fish oil improved mood when compared to placebo, despite an increase in circulating ω-3 polyunsaturated fatty acids." Another study published in October 2007 found that fish oil supplements conferred no additional benefits beyond those conferred by standard treatment.

5.2.2.8 Pregnancy

Omega-3 polyunsaturated fatty acids (commonly found in fish oil) protect against fetal brain injury and promotes fetal and infant brain health. Some studies reported better psycho motor development at 30 months of age in infants whose mothers received fish oil supplements for the first four months of lactation. In addition, five-year-old children whose mothers received modest algae based docosahexaenoic acid supplementation for the first 4 months of breastfeeding performed better on a test of sustained attention. This suggests that docosahexaenoic acid intake during early infancy confers long-term benefits on specific aspects of neurodevelopment.

Docosahexaenoic acid supplementation has also been found to be essential for early visual development of the baby. However, the standard western diet is severely deficient in these critical nutrients. This omega-3 dietary deficiency, a nutrient found in fish oil, is compounded by the fact that pregnant women become depleted in omega-3s, since the fetus uses omega-3s for its nervous system development. Omega-3s are also used after birth if they are provided in breast milk.

In addition, provision of fish oil during pregnancy may reduce an infant's sensitization to common food allergens and reduce the prevalence and severity of certain skin diseases in the first year of life. This effect may persist until adolescence with a reduction in prevalence and/or severity of eczema, hay fever and asthma.

Omega-3 fatty acid supplementation is also beneficial to the mother. It has been shown to prevent pre-term labor and delivery. It is recommended that women who are breastfeeding consume fish oil at least twice a week, although the American Heart Association recommends pregnant and nursing women are to avoiding eating fish with high potential for mercury contaminants including mackerel, shark, or swordfish.

5.2.3 Youtube videos on the Omega 3 Vitamin that I take daily

Nutrilite Salmon Omega 3 (English)

http://www.youtube.com/watch?v=oam00n4aIhI

Uploaded by amwayproducts2020 on Sep 6, 2010

Nutrilite Omega 3- Demo

http://www.youtube.com/watch?v=AWtO8hKjqZE
Uploaded by 84guddu on Jun 23, 2011

If you watch the above videos and follow my weight trend explained earlier in the book there is no doubt that you will realize of the importance of Omega 3 vitamin in your overall health.

5.3 Vitamin B supplement

Here is the standard definition from Wikipedia:

5.3.1 What are B vitamins?

B vitamins are a group of water-soluble vitamins that play important roles in cell metabolism. The B vitamins were once thought to be a single vitamin, referred to as **vitamin B** (much as people refer to vitamin Cor vitamin D). Later research showed that they are chemically distinct vitamins that often coexist in the same foods. In general, supplements containing all eight are referred to as a **vitamin B complex**. Individual B vitamin supplements are referred to by the specific name of each vitamin e.g.

Vitamin B_1 (thiamine)
Vitamin B_2 (riboflavin)
Vitamin B_3 (niacin or niacinamide)
Vitamin B_5 (pantothenic acid)
Vitamin B_6 (pyridoxine, pyridoxal, or pyridoxamine, or pyridoxine hydrochloride)
Vitamin B_7 (biotin)
Vitamin B_9 (folic acid)
Vitamin B_{12} (various cobalamins; commonly cyanocobalamin in vitamin supplements)

5.3.2 What are the health benefits of Vitamins B?

The B vitamins may be necessary to:

- Support and increase the rate of metabolism
- Maintain healthy skin, hair and muscle tone
- Enhance immune and nervous system function
- Promote cell growth and division, including that of the red blood cells that help prevent anemia
- Reduce the risk of pancreatic cancer - one of the most lethal forms of cancer - when consumed in food, but not when ingested in vitamin tablet form.

All B vitamins are water-soluble, and are dispersed throughout the body. Most of the B vitamins must be replenished regularly, since any excess is excreted in the urine.

B vitamins have also been hypothesized to improve the symptoms of attention deficit hyperactivity disorder.

Each of the B vitamins has different safety and usage factors:

- **Vitamin B1** – Easily destroyed by alcohol consumption, caffeine, stress, and smoking. Pregnant women may benefit from slightly higher levels of B1.
- **Vitamin B2** – Absorption or availability is decreased by the use of oral contraceptives, as well as by regular exercise and alcohol consumption. Vegetarians and the elderly may benefit from slightly higher levels of B2.
- **Nicotinic acid (niacin)** – People who exercise regularly, take oral contraceptives, or have a lot of stress in their lives may need slightly higher levels.
- **Vitamin B6** – Pregnant or breastfeeding/lactating women, those who use contraceptives or hormone replacement therapy, and those who use antibiotics regularly may need slightly higher levels. B6 supplementation is also suggested for those who consume alcohol, smoke, and consume protein above recommended levels.
- **Folic acid** – Elderly people and pregnant women may need higher levels, as well as people who consume alcohol or have risk factors associated with heart disease.
- **Vitamin B12** – Strict vegetarians and vegans, along with pregnant and/or lactating women, and those who consume alcohol or smoke may need increased levels.
- **Biotin** – Pregnant women and those who use antibiotics on a long-term basis may need increased levels.
- **Pantothenic acid** – Elderly people and those who take oral contraceptives, as well as those who smoke, or consume alcohol or caffeine may need slightly higher levels.

5.2.3 Youtube videos on the B Complex Vitamin that I take daily

Nutrilite NATURAL - B

http://www.youtube.com/watch?v=RoQyADGCXNY

Uploaded by ultimateeagles on Nov 17, 2008

NUTRILITE Natural B Complex provides a wide spectrum of B vitamins which target nutritional gaps in the daily diet. Many of the B vitamins found in Natural B Complex are naturally derived from yeast. Natural B Complex offers a quick and convenient way to meet your body's demand for this essential vitamin. NUTRILITE Natural B Complex provides a wide variety of benefits:

- Helps to meet the nutritional needs brought on by a stressful life.
- Contains natural minerals to provide a balanced blend of B vitamins, which assist in the release of energy from fats, carbohydrates, and proteins.

NUTRILITE Natural B Complex is used by people working to protect their bodies and/or their emotional balance, as well as women of child-bearing age. **Folic acid**, found in Natural B Complex, is critical for the development of unborn children.

5.4 The website of the World´s best vitamins

http://www.nutrilite.com/ has a lot of sections namely:

- About Nutrilite
- Healthy Lifestyle
- Products
- Health Institute

I wholeheartedly encourage you to browse through the website and breakdown each of the above sections in the corresponding sub-headings.

Likewise it is a critical importance to watch the videos and download podcasts starting with the need for a 9 colour diet on fruits and vegetables. I was an ignorant until I was 44. I had to read specialized books to learn of this critical factor. Their slogan is: Colour yourself healthy.

5.5 The World´s Best Kept Secret

If you look at my professional profile in LinkedIN http://de.linkedin.com/in/jorgezuazola you can see that I have over 2 decades long of experience in well-known publicly traded companies such as Adidas, Fortune Brands, Head in the FMCG sector but also in high-tech such as Nortel and Meta Group.

I am the European equivalent of CPA and hold an MBA Degree from the City of London.

I am fully conversant with Sarbanes-Oxley, US GAAP and IFRS. In other words I am a controls oriented person. I can tell that the current global financial crisis was being created in the Corporate World since the late 90s after the deregulation on the telecom industry in the US.

I am also an author of several books. In my book LinkedIn 100 million users : Leadership is linking up and networking with people I wrote the following:

_____

Why do leading network marketing companies succeed?

In the penultimate chapter of the book I would like to play the devil abdicate role with you. Just in case you still think that because you are in the Corporate World with a well-known company you are safe.

Just in case you think you can retire already very wealthy.

When I read Bill Gates profile in LinkedIn I see that he writes "retired". I envy him. But as I explained earlier his concept did predict the birth of networking giants such as LinkedIn.

However I have also explained earlier that success is not about reinventing the wheel. I know that Linkedin is not a networking marketing company. In fact they are very observant of the rules

http://www.linkedin.com/static?key=user_agreement&trk=hb_ft_userag

29. Participate, directly or indirectly, in the setting up or development of a network that seeks to implement practices that are similar to sales by network or the recruitment of independent home salespeople to the purposes of creating a pyramid scheme or other similar practices.

Therefore we are not talking about pyramid schemes because on the other hand this was already looked into by the Federal Trade Commission in the 70s to conclude it was a remarkable business model. The characteristics of this business model are:

1. *Global Market: Presence in over 80 countries and territories.*

2. *Residual income: Residual income is when you do the work once and you keep getting paid over and over. Networking certainly qualifies on this one. Some networkers have been earning from people they introduced to their networking business some 25 years ago…or more.. This is possible because networking uses the most effective form of advertising: word of mouth. By contrast the traditional business model of Corporations relies on advertising: the problem with advertising is that always half the money is wasted. The irony is that Corporations never know which half is wasted either the first half, or the second half. Or perhaps both.*

3. *Willable: One networking company has third-generation people working for the business and all original lines of sponsorship are still being honored. Is that willable enough for you ? I hope it is because it means that the business you created is transferable to your children when you die. Can you imagine your children not knowing what a job is and having a business as soon as they graduate from the University? I hope you can imagine it and your family*

means a lot.

4. *Duplicatable. The support system of books, tapes, and live events (an open every two weeks, a seminar every month and a convention every quarter) is there to help you to succeed building your network. Tie into the system, and then duplicate yourself by teaching others to do the same.*

5. *Low investment & low maintenance: This may be the best feature of the business. The cost of entry is so low that it is available to virtually anyone. As far as low maintenance, most networkers prefer to work out of their homes, even the hugely successful networkers who can afford to buy a high-rise office building, also work from home. It is not where you work but how you work that counts in this business.*

At present I am not associated with any networking company. However let me paraphrase Jan Vermeiren in his Webinar of March 16th 2010:

- *Linkedin is a networking giant which we can rest our shoulders on and*
- *Adopt a networking attitude to make the 2010 world economy better*

I fully concur with Jan's assessment. I hope you understand why the leading company in network marketing is way ahead of its competitors. Probably also way ahead of your company as their revenues are several (not just 1,2,3,4,5) billions of dollars

Why ? Because they already have their own robust network. Therefore they do not LinkedIn to succeed although of course they have a URL in LinkedIN (like anyone else)

Opinions do not make money, opinions keep people broke

If someone misinformed you about network marketing, then ask yourself two questions:

1. *How did I learn about LinkedIn ?*
2. *Am I bigger or smaller than the person who mentioned/introduced me?*

In my case I am significantly bigger. That is the power of network. The limit to your success is in only in your mind.

I do see LinkedIn hitting 100 million in 1 year from the publication of this book. That is to say, once the 100 million landmark is reached in April 2011 you will have a new window of opportunities ahead of you. The question is: Are you going to ignore it?

The above was written in April 2010. LinkedIn has since then doubled from 65 million to 135 million. It will reach 500 million. Why ? Because of the power of the exponential growth of duplication.

That is why I regard the below company who announced record results for 2010 as the World's Best Kept Secret. They are a privately owned company. They are fully capitalized which ensures that when they open in a new market, their success is guaranteed. That is why they are in over 80 countries and territories around the world.

And when it come to Vitamins it is one of the most audacious leadership stories of life time. The founders Rich De Vos and Jay Van Andel founded Amway based on the Nutrilite model as they were working for that company. A few years later they bought back Nutrilite. This means 100% synergy of business model. This is something which the rest of the business world cannot compete with. The standard Corporate World out there is prisoner of its own model as well as the perceptions from others.

If success is not on your own terms, if it looks good to the world but does not feel good in your soul, it is not success at all. This is what happens to the standard Corporate World companies who are always dependent on outside analysts predictions and earnings calls.

It is very predictable that the below business will exceed 10 billion dollars in 2011. Nutrients (vitamins) was 42 % of the total sales in 2010. It means every year it will get better.

http://www.prnewswire.com/news-releases/amway-parent-grows-to-92-billion-in-2010-116396994.html

Amway Parent Grows to $9.2 Billion in 2010

Strong growth across global markets as direct seller gains market share; brand-building momentum drives 10th sales increase in 11 years

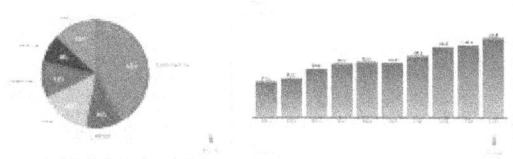

ADA, Mich., Feb. 17, 2011 /PRNewswire/ -- Amway's parent company, Alticor Inc., reported sales exceeding $9.2 billion for the year ended December 31, 2010, a 9.5 percent increase over sales of $8.4 billion in 2009. The 2010 performance results mark Alticor's 10th sales increase in the last 11 years.

The world's second-largest direct selling enterprise, Amway works with more than 3 million distributors who sell the company's branded products, including NUTRILITE® vitamin, mineral and dietary supplements, ARTISTRY® skincare and colour cosmetics, and eSpring® water treatment systems.

The company said that despite an economy recovering from a global recession, 2010 was very solid. "We had a strong year across the map," said chairman Steve Van Andel.

"Amway was able to gain market share in the direct selling industry, and our key product lines improved their competitive position as well."

Said president Doug DeVos: "Awareness of Amway's business opportunity and product brands continues to grow as we invest in brand-building. We believe in the potential of this business, and so do our distributors. We are aiming even higher for 2011."

Alticor also owns Access Business Group, which provides third-party manufacturing and distribution services, and Alticor Corporate Enterprises, a holding company for Amway Hotel Corp., Gurwitch Products, Fulton Innovation and Metagenics. Those subsidiaries also contributed to the year's stronger returns, the company said.

Direct selling business

Amway said growth was fueled by strong 2010 results in China, the company's largest market, as well as healthy gains inIndia, Korea, North America and Latin America. The company, which is privately held, does not generally release individual market sales or disclose profitability.

"Our message of free enterprise and individual opportunity continues to resonate across markets and across cultures," DeVos said. "We're proud to help entrepreneurs take the first step towards business ownership, and to support them with brands that are becoming better known every day."

The company announced that category sales of NUTRILITE approached $4 billion, attributed to overall growth in the category as well as increased visibility for NUTRILITE in 2010. Major campaigns included "Color Yourself Healthy," a global awareness program that promoted the benefits of plant ingredients for optimal health. Global sponsorships focused on major sports teams and well-known athletes continue to build brand awareness for NUTRILITE.

ARTISTRY skin care and cosmetics led beauty category sales for Amway. The company cited a successful launch of ARTISTRY Intensives Renewing Peel, the first product in a new Intensives line of skin care products designed to provide professional results at home. Masstige brand beautycycle™ successfully launched in Europe and Australia, targeted to consumers who are looking for high-quality skin care and cosmetics products containing natural ingredients.

Brand building continues to be a significant focus for Amway around the world. "Our distributors are realizing the benefits of our global investment in building our brands," said DeVos. "It is easier for them to sell products that consumers already know to ask for by name." To increase consumer access to its brands, Amway expanded its physical presences across the globe to complement its direct selling business model.

The company also unveiled a new Amway brand identity in 2010, highlighted by the opening of the Amway Center, home to the National Basketball Association's (NBA) Orlando Magic, which became the first high-profile venue in North America to showcase Amway's new brand identity.

Operationally, the company took steps to evolve into a true global enterprise — leveraging technology to improve supply chain efficiencies, help distributors run their businesses more efficiently and gain consumer insight vital to developing strong customer relationships. Said Van Andel: "We are a global business, with 90 percent of sales outside the U.S., and we are taking necessary steps to support customers worldwide."

Amway One by One Campaign for Children

The Amway One by One Campaign for Children rallies the resources of Amway distributors and employees around the world to make a difference in the lives of children in every market where the company conducts business. Since Amway One by One launched in 2003, it has provided hope and opportunity to 8 million children and donated more than $141 million to children's causes worldwide. The number of employee and distributor volunteer hours logged since 2003 now totals 2.3 million, nearly doubling from a cumulative total of 1.3 million hours reported in 2009.

www.amwayonebyone.com

About Alticor Inc.

Alticor (www.alticor.com) is the parent company of Amway Corporation (www.amway.com), Access Business Group LLC (www.accessbusinessgroup.com) and Alticor Corporate Enterprises. Based in Ada, Michigan (United States), the company offers consumer products and business opportunities, as well as product development, manufacturing and logistics services in more than 80 countries and territories worldwide. With more than 14,000 global employees, Alticor reported 2010 sales exceeding $9.2 billion. Alticor is privately held by the Van Andel and DeVos families, headed by chairman Steve Van Andel and president Doug DeVos, and governed by a board of directors led by members of the two families. For company news, visitglobalnews.amway.com.

SOURCE Alticor Inc.

Back to top

RELATED LINKS

http://www.alticor.com

Based on my worldwide business experience in 30 countries around the world, I have no doubt that this is the World´s Best Kept Business Secret. Those who might disagree should learn this: Humility is the queen of virtues as long as you memorize it and repeat it often. In other words, if you are not well informed, get first-hand information.

CHAPTER 6.GOAL SETTING

"Crystallize your goals. Make a plan for achieving them and set yourself a deadline. Then, with supreme confidence, determination and disregard for obstacles and other people's criticisms, carry out your plan.

Paul Meyer

6.1 Success is goals and everything else is commentary

The heading of this section is based on a quote from Brian Tracy in his books Goals. Whereas I only read the book after achieving my goals on Weight Loss I feel it is the best book out there on goal setting. Here are five powerful reasons why goal setting matters:

1. Meaning

Goal setting motivates you to achieve what you want. Once you know how to set goals, your ability to attach meaning to your deepest desires results in a level of motivation that is greatly overstated but little understood: passion.

Setting goals gives your life more meaning, purpose and passion; surely that makes it worth doing?

2. Time

A person without consciously chosen goals tends to drift from one thing to another. The result? Dissatisfaction caused by a feeling that time has been wasted on things that are either irrelevant, irresponsible or unimportant, as a time management matrix would show.

Well chosen goals mean you spend your time doing things that align with your values -- everything you do has a point and a purpose.

Do you have goals like this yet? Setting goals for yourself will have a positive impact on the quality of your time choices. What you decide to do will possibly scare you, probably challenge you, but definitely mean more to you.

3. Truth

Well chosen goals take you out of your comfort zone. Anything that does this, whether you wanted to do it or not, presents the best opportunity for growth. **Your**growth.

The process may be difficult, even painful, but you discover valuable truths about yourself and the world around you. Your heightened awareness enables you to do something about it.

Once you know, you can grow.

4. Feeling

Yes, the process can be painful, but the journey is often as good as the destination. Why is goal setting important in this respect? The answer is simple and powerful -- it makes **today** better for you. You can remember the past and look forward to, or fear, the future, but you only ever experience 'today'; specifically, this very moment.

Goal setting affects now because it gives you something to look forward to, and that feeling is available this very moment.

At any time, you're free to choose what you think about. Bored, worried or scared? Replace negative thoughts and feelings with something better -- think about what you want.

5. Choice

You choose the direction your life takes -- you assume full responsibility for your actions and their consequences. You're nobody's puppet, or a victim of circumstance. You've always got a choice in what you think, say or do. This is a mindset that many people don't consider. They feel trapped, as if they 'have to'.

It doesn't matter whether your goal is to get something good or leave something bad; accept that you chose everything in your life now, and exercise your freedom to choose from now on.
Do you want to re-commit or move on?

Life makes a habit of habits. It's too easy to do the same things day in, day out without ever really changing. Goals are still set; it's just that they are set to dull the pain of monotony.
Why is goal setting important? Because it injects creativity, promotes growth and ultimately, helps you fulfill your potential.

6.2 The GOSPA Model and the Smart Method

I recommend you Ronnie´s Kagan book The Winning Way: How to Win in life and Enjoy the Journey where he explains the following concepts:

GOSPA Model = Goals Objectives Strategies Plans Actions
SMART = Specific Measurable Aligned Realistic and Time Bound Goals

There is also a LinkedIn Group that I founded called **Success is goals and all else is commentary**
http://www.linkedin.com/groups?about=&gid=4078263&trk=anet_ug_grppro
whose profile is worth reading
A 1979 Harvard Business School study asked graduates:Have you set clear, written goals for your future plans and made plans to accomplish them? Only 3% put written goals and plans. By 1989 those who had clear goals were earning 10 times more than the other 97% of the other graduates all together.

6.3 My Daily Goals Form Monitoring using the concepts of Brian Tracy, Ronnie Kagan and Duke Johnson

A revolution starts with a fundamental change in what we think. It starts with a new way of understanding the world. Understanding becomes belief. And belief changes the way we live and behave for the rest of our lives.

The revolution starts with you – with taking responsibility for your own health. Not that you haven´t wanted to. If you are like most people you just haven´t understood what to do. The result: Your thinking, your beliefs, and your lifestyle are leading you down the path to premature death from chronic diseases. The way to optimal health and longevity involves broad lifestyle changes. It is real revolution, not a phony quick fix. If you join this revolution, you will lose weight – assuming your excessive body fat to start with. But you will use it as a result of achieving a healthy lifestyle, not the other way around. Losing weight will be a healthy side effect of reducing your risk of chronic disease and early death. (Rafael Blanco Elgert, every kilogram you lose, an additional year of life you gain)

GOAL 31.03.11
80.5 kg

1.	To have OHR successfully achieved with 78.4 kg
2.	To literally eliminate any risk of having any sign of obesity i.e. 78.4 kg is my safety valve
3.	To be ideally fit to achieve my espring goals
4.	To be the perfect father for Carmen
5.	To achieve my remaining 25 dreams

The revolution is not about how you look. It is about how you feel, about staying healthy and living longer. You and I aren´t going to look like a twenty something movie star when we are seventy, no matter what we do. But when we are seventy I want us to be healthy, vital and enjoying life.

Yet every day, every hour, we are being sold an idea that is killing us. It is time we all rise up in revolt against the culture that keeps selling it.

Now here is my definition of optimal health: Optimal health is the best health you are capable of, given your past and your generic heritage. You may have made mistakes in your lifestyle up to now. You may not have the best genetics. But the optimal health pathway leads you to the longest, healthiest life possible for you, starting today. We won't all live to the same age. But the earlier you start, the longer and better life you can live.

Every single day since December 2010 I print the goal and have it in front of me visible so that when it comes to eating I remember Shad Helmstetter "It is me who lifts the fork"

CHAPTER 7. NUTRIGENOMICS AND OPTIMAL HEALTH

"Losing weight will be a healthy side effect of reducing your risk of chronic disease and early death "

Duke Johnson

"Every kilogram you lose,
an additional year of life you gain "

Rafael Blanco Elgert

7.1 What is Nutrigenomics ?

Here is the standard definition from Wikipedia:

Nutrigenomics is the science of how nutrients interact with genes. Nutrigenomics is the study of the effects of foods and food constituents on gene expression. It is about how our DNA is transcribed into mRNA and then to proteins and provides a basis for understanding the biological activity of food components. Nutrigenomics has also been described by the influence of genetic variation on nutrition by correlating gene expression or single-nucleotide polymorphisms with a nutrient's absorption, metabolism, elimination or biological effects. By doing so, nutrigenomics aims to develop rational means to optimise nutrition, with respect to the subject's genotype.

By determining the mechanism of the effects of nutrients or the effects of a nutritional regime, nutrigenomics tries to define the causality|relationship between these specific nutrients and specific nutrient regimes (diets) on human health. Nutrigenomics has been associated with the idea of personalized nutrition based on genotype. While there is hope that nutrigenomics will ultimately enable such personalised dietary advice, it is a science still in its infancy and its contribution to public health over the next decade is thought to be major.

Nutrigenomics has been defined as the application of high-throughput genomic tools in nutrition research. It can also be seen as research to provide people with methods and tools who are looking for disease preventing and health promoting foods that match their lifestyles, cultures and genetics.

The term "high throughput tools" in nutrigenomics refers to genetic tools that enable millions of genetic screening tests to be conducted at a single time. When such high throughput screening is applied in nutrition research, it allows the examination of how nutrients affect the thousands of genes present in the human genome. Nutrigenomics involves the characterization of gene products and the physiological function and interactions of these products. This includes how nutrients impact on the production and action of specific gene products and how these proteins in turn affect the response to nutrients.

Throughout the 20th century, nutritional science focused on finding vitamins and minerals, defining their use and preventing the deficiency diseases that they caused. As the nutrition related health problems of the developed world shifted to overnutrition, obesity and type two diabetes, the focus of modern medicine and of nutritional science changed accordingly.

In order to address the increasing incidence of these diet-related-diseases, the role of diet and nutrition has been and continues to be extensively studied. To prevent the development of disease, nutrition research is investigating how nutrition can optimize and maintain cellular, tissue, organ and whole body homeostasis. This requires understanding how nutrients act at the molecular level. This involves a multitude of nutrient-related interactions at the gene, protein and metabolic levels. As a result, nutrition research has shifted from epidemiology and physiology to molecular biology and genetics and nutrigenomics was born.

The emergence and development of nutrigenomics has been possible due to powerful developments in genetic research. Inter-individual differences in genetics, or genetic variability, which have an effect on metabolism and on phenotypes were recognized early in nutrition research, and such phenotypes were described. With the progress in genetics, biochemical disorders with a high nutritional relevance were linked to a genetic origin. Genetic disorders which cause pathological effects were described. Such genetic disorders include the polymorphism in the gene for the hormone Leptin which results in gross obesity. Other gene polymorphisms were described with consequences for human nutrition. The folate metabolism is a good example, where a common polymorphism exists for the gene that encodes the methylene-tetrahydro-folate reductase (MTHFR).

It was realized however, that there are possibly thousands of other gene polymorphisms which may result in minor deviations in nutritional biochemistry, where only marginal or additive effects would result from these deviations. The tools to study the physiological impact were not available at the time and are only now becoming available enabling the development of nutrigenomics. Such tools include those that measure the transcriptome - DNA microarray, Exon array, Tiling arrays, single nucleotide polymorphism arrays and genotyping. Tools that measure the proteome are less developed. These include methods based on gel electrophoresis, chromatography and mass spectrometry. Finally the tools that measure the metabolome are also less developed and include methods based on nuclear magnetic resonance imaging and mass spectrometry often in combination with gas and liquid chromatography.

7.2 Youtube videos on Nutrigenomics

The New Science of Nutrigenomics Unveiled

http://www.youtube.com/watch?v=Prwds4eVEiA

Dr. Mark Hyman takes you one step further by explaining exciting recent research from Dr. Dean Ornish that shows exactly why this is possible -- through the new science of nutrigenomics. For more, please seehttp://www.ultrawellness.com/blog.

Uploaded by ultrawellness on Jan 10, 2008

Dr. Perricone Discusses Nutrigenomics

http://www.youtube.com/watch?v=I57PJRHxoWA

Uploaded by DrPerricone on Aug 31, 2010

Whose book is Forever Young: The Science of Nutrigenomics for Glowing, Wrinkle-Free Skin and Radiant Health at Every Age

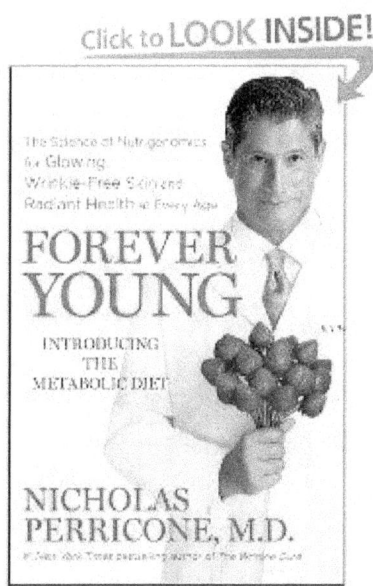

Which you can order at http://www.amazon.com/Forever-Young-Science-Nutrigenomics-Wrinkle-Free/dp/B005OHS9YI/ref=sr_1_4?ie=UTF8&qid=1323517954&sr=8-4

As the video says there is a special discount. In my case I only paid 3.59 Euros to get it.

Dr Duke Johnson, Nutrilite

http://www.youtube.com/watch?v=2thraihi-KA

Uploaded by insider201283 on Mar 21, 2009

Dr Duke Johnson Medical Director, Nutrilite Center of Optimal Health, talks about the benefits of a plant based diet and organic, plant based supplements in achieving optimal health

Dr. Duke on Optimal Health

http://www.youtube.com/watch?v=TfMgq6z3aQs

Uploaded by greenlitebites on Nov 16, 2009

You really want to see the above video specially when Dr Duke Johnson talks about the steroids taken by sports men and Hollywood actors.

His book is the Bible of Optimal Health

The Optimal Health Revolution: How Inflammation Is the Root Cause of the Biggest Killers and How the Cutting-edge Sceince of Nutrigenomics Can Transform Your Long-term Health

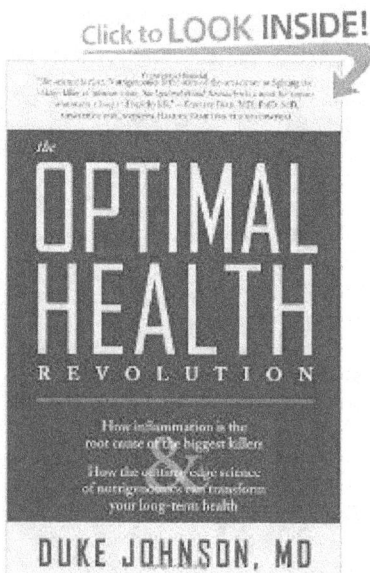

http://www.amazon.com/gp/offer-listing/1933771828/ref=tmm_pap_used_olp_sr?ie=UTF8&qid=1323518332&sr=1-1&condition=used

Not ordering this book can be the biggest mistake of your life. I can see that in amazon you can order for as little as 0.88 $ depending always on which retailer has it on offer.

7.3 Linkedin Group on Nutrigenomics

LinkedIn has a Group called Nutrigenomics http://www.linkedin.com/groups?about=&gid=1900547&trk=anet_ug_grppro which was founded by Danijel Stojkovic Researcher http://si.linkedin.com/in/danijelstojkovic at University of Nova Gorica in Slovenia.

The group focuses on nutritional genomics, personalized nutrition and other next-generation nutrition related topics. The group is open to scientific, technical, commercial and managerial professionals. Other genomics and/or nutrition enthusiasts are welcome as well.

The Group has professionals with an interest in Nutrition but from all walks of life and all parts of the world from Switzerland to the US from Canada to New Zealand and from Slovenia to Holland.

In the Group you can find the following relevant topics:

- Genetic engineering and biotechnology

- Microalgae food application

- Podcasts of interviews with experts

- Article reviews on genes

- How to apply nutrigenomics for measuring metabolic health

- Keys to weight loss

and many others

7.4 OHR Literature

OHR is now my health acronym. Exactly as I did with SW from Ronnie Kagan I have now called my acronym OHR which stands for Optimal Health Revolution. Whereas I only read the book from Duke Johnson between December 2010 and January 2011 (when most of my weight loss targets had already been achieved) I must admit that this book was my final wake-up call on health.

Throughout this section I will be sharing a number of key concepts for you. However I would urge to buy the book from Dr. Duke Johnson and apply it to the letter. As you shall see below I myself have plenty to apply and improve on.

7.4.1 Obesity and Chronic inflammation

Dr Duke Johnson says that the World Health Organization (WHO) states that there is an epidemic of obesity occurring around the world, to the extent that there may now be more obese people in the world than starving people. On balance, that is a good thing. It is a sign of real social, political and economic progress that more people are dying from excessive junk-food consumption that from starvation. But both extremes are forms of malnutrition, and the nutritional deficiencies of the affluent also take millions of lives prematurely even if not as rapidly as starvation.

He further adds that the WHO states also that there is an epidemic of type 2 diabetes (previously referred to as adult-onset diabetes) occurring around the world. Expenditures for treating type 2 diabetes have quadrupled in Japan over the last ten years and have doubled in most other industrialized nations.

I did not doubt any of what Doctor Johnson wrote. However as a conservative auditor and controller I also research on the WHO website which has a section called

Controlling the global obesity epidemic

Which includes two major topics

1. The challenge

    At the other end of the malnutrition scale, obesity is one of today's most blatantly visible – yet most neglected – public health problems. Paradoxically coexisting with undernutrition, an escalating global epidemic of overweight and obesity – "globesity" – is taking over many parts of the world. If immediate action is not taken, millions will suffer from an array of serious health disorders.

    Obesity is a complex condition, one with serious social and psychological dimensions, that affects virtually all age and socioeconomic groups and threatens to overwhelm both developed and developing countries. In 1995, there were an estimated 200 million obese adults worldwide and another 18 million under-five children classified as overweight. As of 2000, the number of obese adults has increased to over 300 million. Contrary to conventional wisdom, the obesity epidemic is not restricted to industrialized societies; in developing countries, it is estimated that over 115 million people suffer from obesity-related problems.

Generally, although men may have higher rates of overweight, women have higher rates of obesity. For both, obesity poses a major risk for serious diet-related noncommunicable diseases, including diabetes mellitus, cardiovascular disease, hypertension and stroke, and certain forms of cancer. Its health consequences range from increased risk of premature death to serious chronic conditions that reduce the overall quality of life.

2. The response: making healthy choices easy choices

WHO began sounding the alarm in the 1990s, spearheading a series of expert and technical consultations. Public awareness campaigns were also initiated to sensitize policy-makers, private sector partners, medical professionals and the public at large. Aware that obesity is predominantly a "social and environmental disease", WHO is helping to develop strategies that will make healthy choices easier to make. In collaboration with the University of Sydney (Australia), WHO is calculating the worldwide economic impact of overweight and obesity. It is also working with the University of Auckland (New Zealand) to analyse the impact that globalization and rapid socioeconomic transition have on nutrition and to identify the main political, socioeco-nomic, cultural and physical factors which promote obesogenic environments.

Dr Duke Johnson further backs up WHO findings with his participants of his program from China, Malaysia, India, Thailand, Japan, Russia, Korea., Hong Kohn, Brazil, Argentina, Venezuela, Great Britain, Germany, Austria, Italy, Poland or the US they all had the same risk factors for major chronic diseases and were beginning to show evidence of these diseases. With technological advances, we have begun to adopt very similar lifestyles globally.

He argues that

1. We must have the courage and patience to forge a new pathway to optimal health. Our global problem with chronic diseases did not develop overnight, nor they will disappear overnight.

2. A risk factor is any lifestyle component or biological trait that increases the risk of a chronic disease.

3. Inflammation is the cause of heart diseases and cancer, as well as many other chronic diseases.

4. Almost every aspect of our "normal" industrialized lifestyles stimulates our immune systems to become chronically overactive. The over-activity results in a chronic release of the molecules that cause the inflammation. Until we focus our effort on this root cause, we will have only marginal success at controlling the individual diseases that pop up from its unseen roots.

To my mind, it is very clear that Duke Johnson concurs with José Manuel González Griego my General Practitioner in Frankfurt (featured in the front page of this book) that obesity is an illness. José Manuel rang me up on an icy December 2010 evening to have a coffee here in Germany. It was one of his calls without having arranged a meeting. He caught me having dinner but I showed up at the local coffee bar. To his astonishment I showed up with Duke Johnson's book as well as that of Dale Carnegie (How to Stop Worrying and Start Living).

José Manuel was impressed with the outlay of the book from Duke Johnson and wanted to borrow it from me. I refused. My argument was this one based on Napoleon Hill

"The starting point of all achievement is desire. Keep this constantly in mind. Weak desires bring weak results, just as a small fire makes a small amount of heat."

In March 2011 I went to see José Manuel at his office when I was 80.5kg. He was happy but a bit jealous as he was 91 kg. I went to see him to do the tests that Duke Johnson advises for a person of my age. José Manuel was scared that something would show up in the tests. The results were immaculate. I was confident they would be. I told him that he loved the book cover page that all the causes of any disease are an excessive inflammation.

As always the standard definition of wikipedia is worth reading. Obesity is a medical condition in which excess body fat has accumulated to the extent that it may have an adverse effect on health, leading to reduced life expectancy and/or increased health problems. Body mass index (BMI), a measurement which compares weight and height, defines people as overweight (pre-obese) if their BMI is between 25 and 30 kg/m^2, and obese when it is greater than 30 kg/m^2.

Obesity increases the likelihood of various diseases, particularly heart disease, type 2 diabetes, obstructive sleep apnea, certain types of cancer, and osteoarthritis. Obesity is most commonly caused by a combination of excessive food energy intake, lack of physical activity, and genetic susceptibility, although a few cases are caused primarily by genes, endocrine disorders, medications or psychiatric illness. Evidence to support the view that some obese people eat little yet gain weight due to a slow metabolism is limited; on average obese people have a greater energy expenditure than their thin counterparts due to the energy required to maintain an increased body mass.

Dieting and physical exercise are the mainstays of treatment for obesity. Moreover, it is important to improve diet quality by reducing the consumption of energy-dense foods such as those high in fat and sugars, and by increasing the intake of dietary fiber. To supplement this, or in case of failure, anti-obesity drugs may be taken to reduce appetite or inhibit fat absorption. In severe cases, surgery is performed or an intragastric balloon is placed to reduce stomach volume and/or bowel length, leading to earlier satiation and reduced ability to absorb nutrients from food.

Obesity is a leading preventable cause of death worldwide, with increasing prevalence in adults and children, and authorities view it as one of the most serious public health problems of the 21st century. Obesity is stigmatized in much of the modern world (particularly in the Western world), though it was widely perceived as a symbol of wealth and fertility at other times in history, and still is in some parts of the world.

In other words José Manuel is right but he has not done the transition to stop taking everything which is inflammatory as I shall explain later. This takes us to the next topics.

7.4.2 Why is Chronic Excessive Inflammation the Monster ?

According to Dr. Duke Johnson inflammation is

1. A non-specific protective immune system response to cell injury or irritation that is characterized by capillary enlargement, attraction of white blood cells to the area, redness, local swelling, and partial reduction of normal cell function.

2. The star player, the big scorer, on our opponent's team. Our game plan for optimal health has to be built around it.

He argues that there is a great deal of interaction between the risk factors for obesity and those for all other chronic disease. This is why it is imperative that we help you change your total lifestyle. It is the only way to treat the underlying problem, the only way to achieve optimal health.

He further backs up his advice with the proven fact that problems pile up faster that we can deal with them and we are overwhelmed – and the result is that we become emotionally inflamed. The same thing can happen with our immune system, except that the inflammation isn't figurative, its response can damage innocent tissue, just as out-of-control emotions can damage relationships with colleagues and family. In order to protect our health we need to control the causes of excess inflammation.

He concludes that dramatic changes in our lifestyles over the last several decades have caused the steep rise in chronic inflammation. These lifestyle changes will have different effects on the bodies of different people because of our generic differences, but we have been affected to some degree.

He finalizes with "I don't want to take what I am saying about inflammation on faith. I want you to understand the science."

In other sections of his book Dr. Johnson comes to say that every day we are sold an idea which is killing us. 2 months later I read the book Everyone communicates a few connect by John C. Maxwell who also comes to say the same thing from a different perspective i.e. we get bombarded by e-mails, TV commercials, Radio slogans, Press advertisements which kill us.

If you think I am being dogmatic here, let me share this experience with you. I happened to watch the Spanish King's Cup final on Soccer in the German Television. During the break the German TV broadcasted ads on beer and sausages. My stomach ached watching those ads. Why ? Because I then thought of what both Duke Johnson and Maxwell say. I had been eating the famous German sausages all my life and they are not any good for my health. Equally drinking beer is drinking alcohol. Whereas I have never been a heavy drinker since I read that alcohol is in Duke Johnson's list of items to be avoided at all times, I have promised myself that I will never drink a glass of wine or a glass of beer no matter what the people might do.

7.4.3 17 steps for reducing chronic inflammation

Duke Johnson outlines a 17 step plan for reducing chronic inflammation. Whereas to read all the details of what he recommends you need to read his book by the letter I can outline how I had taken some of the steps already in my quest to defeat obesity forever.

1. **Reduce the risk factors for chronic disease:** This is the most important effective step you can take according to Dr. Johnson who lists these risk in detail in 4 chapters (9 to 12) of his book. In my case it was very clear: I was obese for over a decade and had no choice: If I did not beat obesity I would have a risk factor on my health permanently.

2. **Consume natural anti-inflammatories like omega 3:** Duke Johnson points out that Modern diets have turned away from healthy oils like omega-3 which is a natural anti-inflammatory, in favor of cheap, inflammatory oils like corn oil. When I read that the first thing I did was to invest 600 Euros in a state of the art cook technology called I cook. This coupled with a first class Italian olive oil and the Omega 3 vitamin I was taking since October 2010 meant that I had taken step 2 correctly.

3. **Exercise**: Here Duke Johnson makes the point that research has shown that exercise is also associated with reduction of inflammation. Even simple walks near your residence, playing with your children in a park etc. is exercise and will be beneficial. You don't have to join a club to participate in exercise that will reduce your risk of chronic disease. Even leisure-time walking has been shown to reduce inflammation and adding suplementation provides greater anti-inflammatory benefits.

In my case this step had been applied as follows

Walk 20 minutes after lunch, 30 minutes after dinner and 1 hour before going to bed
Jog 25 minutes at least 5 days a week

I will refer to this later on in the book.

4. **Take a good multivitamin/multimineral** as he describes in chapter 8 of his book. In my case I had already done the homework required via Double X Multivitamin Complex

5. **Reduce saturated, trans and omega-6 fatty acids in your diet. Duke Johsonn says that**

   -these are the fats associated with inflammation.
   -Darkmeats and partially hydrogenated oils contain omega-6.
   -Oils that are higher in omega-6 are corn, safflower, cottonseed, sunflower, peanut, sesame, grapeseed, primrose, and soybean oils (although soybean oild has some omega-3). The only oils we recommend are canol and virgin oliver oils.
   As stated earlier I only cook with a high quality Italian olive oil.

   It makes a tremendous difference because before I was cooking with sunflower oil.

6. **Take reasonable levels of antioxidant/anti-inflamatory supplements**, especially those that rich in phytonutrients (like resveratrol) from concentrated food sources. Antioxidants have been shown to reduce inflammation. Among the nutrients or components that have been shown to reduce inflammation are coenzyme Q10, lycopene, magnesium, glucosamine, and quercentin.

   When I read this recommendation from Duke Johnson I was fast enough to order Coenyzme Q10. I felt guilty but I admitted my ignorance. Someone who is aged 65 had been asking me to buy Coenzyme for him for years. In my ignorance I never asked for. Now I can see why

7. **Even 7 to 9 servings of fruits and vegetables per day.** Duke Johnson makes the following clear points:

   -There is no substitute for eating vegetables and fruits. They are loaded with natural antioxidants and phytonutrients that reduce inflammation.
   -For example one group of plant chemicals or phytonutrients has both antioxidant and anti-inflammatory qualities.

-Examples in this group and good sources are quercertin (onions, kale, blueberries, broccoli and tea) flavenols (green tea and cocoa), hesperatin (tomatoes and oranges). flavones (parsley, celery) isoflavones (soy) and anthocyanins (grapes, beans, onions, and berries).

-Hopefully you can see why there is no substitute for 7 to 9 daily servings of fruits and vegetables of different colours.

Later on he comes to say that 9 better than 7. Since then I have invariable taken 9 daily servings of fruits and vegetables. I will explain that later on. But basically any time I have a major meal I make sure that both a mixed salad and cooked vegetables are part of the menu. I need to get better with colours.

8. **Avoid process foods:** These are the foods laden with high frucose corn syrup, partially hydrogenated oils, and other chemicals. The more chemicals added to your food via processing, the greater your chance of chronic inflammation according to Dr. Johnson.

   Since I read this I am not taking any processed food. To me this now includes a piece of bread or even a youghourt or an ice cream. When I see José Manuel visiting me with an ice cream in my gym I cannot accept it. He is my doctor but I tell him it is wrong to eat it.

9. **Avoid fast food:** Studies have shown that eating fast food increases the inflammatory response in the body. This is most likely related to the quality of fast food due to its cheap ingredients that are inflammatory and mentioned elsewhere.

   Needless to say that I do not recall the last time I have eaten at fast food restaurant. I do not recall the last time I have eaten a burger.

10. **Eat organically grown and raised fruits, vegetables, meats and diary products.** Duke Johnson says not to forget to wash the organic produce, though, because it can still have bacteria on the outside. There are still chemicals that can build up and cause chronic inflammation he argues.

    I always washed all the fruits but now I even take care of washing them with a special

11. **Eat carbohydrates with a low glycemic lead:** Duke Johnson says that this means that they are low in simple sugars because the higher the sugar load in your diet the greater your risk of elevated CRP.

    Here is where I have been unable to do the CRP test with José Manuel yet. I have now seen a friend who has a BMI of 16, his secret is not having any sugar.

I need to learn this to be optimal.

12. **Follow the nutrigenomics guideline explained in Chapter 4 of his book.** All recommendations in this book – including Appendix on medical tests to perform- are all based upon the best nutrigenomics scientific information.

I passed the tests of my age without a problem but need to get perfect on this

13. **Take low dose aspirin or another anti-inflammatory:** Established medicine has recommended aspirin to patients for years to reduce the risk of having heart attacks because of ifs tendency to reduce clotting in the arteries. However we found to our surprise a few years ago that people who have taken aspirin for many years also have a reduced risk of colon cancer. The aspirin helped reduce the inflammation that can lead to chronic diseases in addition to heart disease.

This recommendation from Duke Johnson is very interesting. However I have not put this in practice yet. I need to discuss it with my General Practitioner.

14. **Take adequate amounts of vitamins D**. Vitamin D supplementation has been shown to be associated with reduced inflammation. Vitamin D and calcium together have shown to also reduce inflammation.

I now take Calcium Magnesium and Vitamin D suplemments

15. **Get adequate sleep**: Inadequate sleep causes inflammation.

Great advice from Dr Johnson. I have now made a simple calculation. 24 hours time 7 days a week comes to 168 hours. If I sleep 7 hours a day I spend 30% of the time (168) sleeping. Less than that is no good. More than that is no good. Thus if I go to bed at 23 hours I find it hard to get up at 5 am. I therefore know that by 22 hours I must be in bed. Likewise Saturday and Sundays have to be a normal day. I have to wake up early to be in motion. Otherwise Monday I start with laziness. Which is no good.

16. **Reduce salt intake**: High salt intake increases inflammation

I take no salt at all in my meals.

17. **Talk to your doctor**: If you rigorously follow the first 16 steps, you often won´t need medication.

I take no medication whatsoever for the amazement of my doctor José Manuel. If I get sick I get angry because I have read from Dr. Johnson that my urine has to be between white and yellow and my defecation light brown. Other than that it means that what I have eaten was not right. Or that, as we said earlier in the book, I have not drunk the right amount of water. Remember, you are what you drink.

7.4.3 My actions on the 8 Pillars of Optimal Health

Duke Johnson gives all of us a fundamental advise "Ask anybody for directions and he or she becomes an expert, regardless of qualification. This applies to both navigation and advice about your health. Everybody has an opinion. And you get bad advice. "

This is probably the best advice Duke Johnson gives us. I have had all my life time wasters telling me what to do on health. They include of course members of my family. Back in 2007 I was weighting almost 120 kg (264.5 lb) and my blood pressure had a minimum of 110. All the family members who were surrounding me in Marbella, Spain were giving me a hard time. Their advice was ill founded. The confused my GP telling her that I had anxiety. I ended up having the wrong prescription without the blessing of José Manuel in Frankfurt. As a result I had to take a counter treatment under his guidance, simply because the wrong prescriptions had created a dependence on benzos when all I needed was to lose weight.

Once again it proved clear what Duke Johnson says. Those who are close to you have no clue on optimal health. Yet you listen to them. Once again what Shad Helsmtetter says on his videos "From the moment you are born you are told…" proved correct.

That is why I have the OHR acronym memorized. Because Duke Johnson says

"Optimal Health means having the best health possible given your genetic heritage, personal history, and environment. Ideally, the foundation for optimal health should be started before we are conceived."

These are the 8 pillars of Optimal Health according to Dr. Duke Johnson and this is how I apply them

Pillar #1 : Reduce Your Risk Factor for Chronic Diseases
A risk factor is any lifestyle or biological quality or characteristics that can increase your likelihood of developing a disease.

My Action: I no longer perform 100% travelling jobs which require me to live out of a suitcase because then I cannot control the ideal nutrition

Pillar #2: Exercise

Duke Johnson says that most sedentary folks argue they don´t have time to exercise. People can´t see how exercise can possibly fit into their lives or their budgets. Here are some examples of the exercise of daily living from Doctor Johnson:

- Take stairs instead of escalators or elevators. If you work on the 50th floor take the elevator to 48th.
- Park on the outer edges of parking lots and walk the rest of the way
- Carry your luggage instead of using rollers
- Buy a walk-behind lawn mower instead of a riding one-and don't pay some kid to push it
- If you take a train or bus to work, get off a few blocks early and walk the rest of the day
- Take a walk with your spouse or play outdoors with your kids.
- Take dancing lessons. I know of people who have lost 20-plus pounds (10-plus kg) after they joined a dance class and are having a great time maintaining that weight loss.

He concludes with this tip "Add the exercise of daily living to your life. It takes very little time and can dramatically reduce your risk of chronic disease".

My action: Swimming 5 days a week at 6.30 am, walking always after each major meal. Jogging 5 times a week and body building in the Gym 3 times a week.

Pillar #3: Good Macronutrition

According to Duke Johnson, the Institute of Medicine recommends that the ranges of macronutrients in adult's daily diets be:

- 45-65 percent carbohydrates
- 20-35 percent fats
- 10-35 percent proteins

A balanced diet must also include good daily sources of fiber

My action: I always take pasta in the meals. I always drink a glass of protein powder every day. I always have plenty of lettuce in my meals and fiber supplements in my list of vitamins

Pillar #4: Good Micronutrition

If macronutrition relates to the bulk of your diet, micronutrition is the stuff that comes in tiny but critical amounts in our food. This includes not only vitamins and minerals but also phytonutrients. The prefix "phyto" derives from the Greek word for plant. Phytonutrients are active nutrients found in plants that are not defined as vitamins or minerals – for example, lycopene.

My action: I take all the Nutrilite vitamins in the recommended doze i.e. including the concentrate of fruits and vegetable to ensure I get all the colours.

Pillar #5: Mind, Spirit and Positive Attitude

We have known for years that happy and hopeful people are generally healthier and longer-lived than the perennially depressed, angry, fear and pessimistic. This phenomenon is miraculous: Recent scientific research has finally been able to pinpoint the physiological cause and effect: Depression triggers two hormonal pathways that worsen our overall health.

My action: Application of the golden hour by the book i.e. get up at 5 am and spend 1 hour reading. I read this in 2010 in Brian Tracy´s focal point and gives me full mind, spirit and positive attitude.

Pillar # 6: Adequate Rest

Of our 8 pillars, this one may need the most shoring up. People in modern civilizations do not get enough sleep. **What is the optimal amount of sleep to get ?** Between 7 and 8 hours of sleep appears to be the best for the vast majority of adults.

My action: 7 hours times 7 days is 49 hours which divided by 168 hours gives us 30% of our time sleeping. That is more than enough.

Pillar # 7: Good Medical Care

Duke Johnson recommends regular check-ups as outlined in the appendices of his book

My action: All what applies to a man in his mid 40s has been scheduled. Instead of going to the doctor with fear I now go with proactivity. I am asking for tests all the time.

Pillar # 8: Healthy Environment and Good Hygiene

Duke Johnson says that air pollution is associated with many upper respiratory diseases, cancers and an increased risk of heart disease. You need to be very careful of bottled water because it may not be safer than your own tap water. There are some good bottled water companies but a lot is just tap water, bought from municipal water companies, marked about 10,000 percent and labeled with a picture of pristine, bubbling spring. Another important of this pillar is hygiene. Monogamy is a great defense against a variety of diseases. This may seem like common sense, but optimal health is very difficult to maintain if you frequently expose yourself to the possibly infected body fluids of others.

My action: I only drink espring water. I am divorced and will not marry somebody again until my daughter Carmen and I have jointly achieved financial independence.

7.4.4 My score on Duke Johnson tips for reducing stress, inflammation, overall risk factors and cancer factors

What follows is a series of items listed in Duke Johnson´s game plan and how I have personally adhered to it both when I started my quest to defeat obesity and after interiorizing the acronym OHR

Game plan for reducing stress

1. Proper nutrition
2. Day planners and time-management systems
3. Enough sleep
4. Exercise
5. Music
6. Meditation
7. Escape

My actions:I do apply 1, 2, 3, 4 and 6. Music CDs. I need to get better on point 7

Dietary supplementary´s role in the reduction of inflammation 13 rules

1. More is not better
2. Natural does not mean safe
3. Buying something from a health food store does not guarantee it is healthy
4. Avoid supplements that contain multiple herbs
5. Check how a supplement is made
6. Choose food over synthetic chemicals
7. Opt for organic
8. Do some research
9. Money isn´t everything
10. Be cautious of Aryuvedic products
11. Listen to the right people
12. Beware of drug interactions
13. Get Smart

My actions: I apply all the rules by the book

Risk factors of Major Chronic Diseases Defeating Your Heart Disease, Your Toughest Opponent Let us get starting on beating your heart disease, by going through the risk factors 1 by 1 and talking about how you can defend yourself against them

1. Family History and genetic predisposition
2. Diabetes
3. Smoking
4. High blood pressure
   He says more than 115/75 is a risk
5. Lack of exercise
6. Obesity
7. Elevated lipids
8. Not enough fruits and vegetables
9. Depression
10. Stress
11. Lack of intrinsic faith
12. Homocysteine

13. Hypothyroidism

14. Lack of omega-3 in your diet

15. Elevated inflammation. CRP (C-Reactive Protein) (ask your doctor about a high sensitive CRP test)

My actions: I just need to take the CRP test with José Manuel. However point 4 denotes my personal satisfaction. Back in 2007 I had minimum blood pressure of 110. Now I know that around 115 has to be my maximum.

Checkmating Cancer. The 16 Risk Factors of Cancer

1. Family History and genetic predisposition
2. Smoking
3. Lack of exercise
4. Obesity
5. Stress
6. Animal fat
7. Not enough fruits and vegetables
8. Excessive Alcohol
9. High salt intake
10. Pollution
11. Smoke or grilled foods
12. Excessive sunlight
13. Certain infections (HPV test)
14. Vitamin D deficiency
15. Inflammation
16. Insulin resistance and type 2 diabetes

My actions: All of them controlled perhaps discuss with José Manuel the tests

7.4.5 Calculations for Body Fat. BMI Weight and Hips and Formula

BMI formula using the metric system
(Body weight in Kilograms, height in meters)
Weight/(Height * Height)

BMI is used to classify body weights in 4 general categories. For adults of European descent, it breaks out this way:

Under 19 = underweight
19 to 24.9 = normal
25 to 29.9 = overweight
30 or above = obese

$$82,1$$
$$1,81 \quad 1,81 \qquad 3,2761$$

82,1   3,2761   25,06029

81,6
1,81   1,81   3,2761
            81,6   3,2761   24,90766

The two above calculations represent NOT THE IDEAL BMI but the frontier between what can be consider normal and overweight. This was highlighted by a Spanish nutritionist in my homeland of Bilbao in November 2011. Here is translation for you.

_____

—

Obesity causes cancer
A nutritionist today opens the lecture series "To live better," organized by the Clinic of Navarra Bilbao. Body mass index is a number obtained by dividing the number of kilos you weigh by height in meters squared. If the number exceeds 25, is already talking about overweight

Being overweight is closely linked to cancer. Obese people have higher risk of cancer disease, because there is a "very direct"relationship between obesity and the occurrence of certain tumors. 'Cancers are not caused by a single cause, but due to a very wide range of factors. To say that obesity is more important than others in the emergence of a tumor disease would be a fallacy, but is very involved in the outset of cancer is absolutely true. Any treatment for obesity should be considered, therefore, as one more element to consider in the prevention of neoplastic disease, "says the director of the Department of Endocrinology and Nutrition, University Hospital of Navarra (CUN), Francisco Javier Salvador , which will offer a conference today in Bilbao on 'How to combat the epidemic of obesity and its complications'.

Salvador's talk lecture opens health clinics organized by Pamplona in Bilbao this month. The program, organized under the motto "To live better," plans to hold three speeches, including today, which will take place on three consecutive Thursdays, from half past seven pm in the auditorium of BBVA Bilbao (Gran Vía, 1).
The specialist Navarro argues that there is insufficient evidence to conclude that obesity is "intimately connected" with cancers that have "a hormonal basis," such as breast, ovarian and endometrial cancer in women and colon, prostate, kidney and bladder in males. "No statistics are devastating, but the relationship is undeniable," to the extent that, according to the expert, "if one studies the prevalence of these tumors in the obese population, find, because there is already work on the issue, which is clearly higher than non-obese population. '

Adipose tissue, as has been discovered in recent years, is not inert, but, quite the contrary, is a living tissue, where cells reproduce very quickly, in a "spectacular". This situation, coupled with the onset of hormonal changes and phenomena such as the emergence of resistance to insulin in the blood, significantly favors the development of these tumors.
Sleep Apnea
Cancer may be the most feared disease associated with overweight and obesity, but not the only one. Both health problems, which are the same in varying degrees, are

directly related to the development of cardiovascular disease, hypertension, diabetes ... The complete relationship with sleep apnea, a condition that according to the latest research is much more common than previously thought. Over 80% of people with a BMI less than 35 have breathing problems while sleeping so severe that they can kill.

The BMI is a number obtained by dividing the number of kilos you weigh by height in meters squared. If the number exceeds 25, we are already talking overweight. The interruption of breathing during sleep, a common disorder not only linked to overweight, is produced for seconds or minutes, long enough to cause a heart attack."It's deadly serious, which can be prevented largely through weight control," says Javier Salvador

___

Therefore 25 is the measure which can never exceed

That is why my success was 80.5 kg (177.1 lbs) because then

```
80,5
1,81      1,81    3,2761
          80,5    3,2761   24,5719
```

The above gives us 24.5 and yet....the safeguard measure is 24

```
78,6
1,81      1,81    3,2761
          78,6    3,2761  23,99194
```

Which means that I have to weight 78.6 kg (172.9 lbs) to be away from the risk zone. You see whereas what I did was remarkable it is still far from perfect. I hope you get the message. 25 BMI is the limit you cannot surpass. 24 is the ideal and optimal measure to avoid further complications.

With regards Waist / hips should equal 0.95 or less for men

And finally the complete formula is

Formula
(BMI/25) + (% body fat /27) + (waist-to-hip-ratio/0,85) / 3 =

BCoR Scores	Men	Women
Underweight	Less than 0.64	Less than 0.74
Ideal (low risk)	0.64 -0.84	0.74-0.87
Normal	0.85 – 1.0	0.88- 1.0
Increased risk	1.0-1.13	1.0 1.13
Significant risk	More than 1.13	More than 1.13

Which means I still have to take the body fat test with José Manuel (and the CRP test) to reach the ideal (low risk) of 0.64 to 0.84.

This reminds me of the leadership principle that success is a journey not a destination. This is something that Vicente del Bosque, Spain's soccer national coach says always in very humble terms.

7.4.6 The causes of obesity and the 25 steps for optimal health

Obesitiy is a disease whose primary behavioral causes are
1. Ignorance
2. Excess calories
3. Obsession over fats and carbs
4. Lack of exercise
5. Narrow focus
6. The TV, the PC and the VWW
7. Coping with stress by eating
8. Snack foods
9. Feeding our emotions
10. Quitting on your new lifestyle
11. Restaurant food, both fast and slow
12. Genetic predisposition
13. Lack of adequate sleep

I have dealt with all the causes, I need to discipline myself a bit more with regards to the timing spent in front of a PC

Twenty five easy steps to Optimal Health
1. Eat more fruit and vegetables
2. Quit or decrease smoking
3. Eat more whole grains:
4. Get help for depression or stress:
5. Calculate your BMI, waist-to-hip ratio and percentage body fat
6. Calculate how many calories you need:
7. Learn how to estimate your calorie intake
8. Wear sunscreen:
9. Eat carbohydrates with low glycemic index
10. Take basic supplements:

11. Kick the fad habit:.
12. Exercise your religious faith:
13. Avoid high fructose corn syrup
14. Get enough rest
15. Use only canola and extra- virgin olive oil
16. Eat organic foods as much as possible.
17. Decrease alcohol use, preferably to zero
18. Get more omega-3 in your diet and (if cleared by your doctor) through supplementation
19. Reduce exposure to contagious diseases especially sexually transmitted diseases
20. See your doctor to be checked for recommendations
21. Cut back on processed foods, including fast food and snacks
22. Move your body more
23. Reduce your exposure to chemicals
24. Reduce consumption of dark meats especially beef, pork and processed meats because of their omega-6 and chemical content
25. Get generic testing: Ask your doctor about generic tests

I still need to do the percentage body fat calculation as well as the calories intakes. I need my GP José Manuel to help me on this.

7.4.7 The medical tests for men of my age i.e. 40 to 50

This is what Doctor Duke Johnson recommends:

1. Complete physical exam yearly, including urianalyisis and blood testing with CBC, chemistry panel, fasting glucose, hs-C-reactive protein, homocysteine, VAP cholesterol panel, liver panel, fasting insulin and omega-3 levels

2. Digital rectal exam yearly for prostate and rectal abnormalities

3. Stool for occult blood yearly

4. Complete eye exam by ophthalmologist

5. Yearly prostate-specific amtigen (PSA)

6. Baseline exercise treadmill and every three years depending on risk

7. Bone density every three years (more frequently if problems are already present)

7.4.8 Food contents to avoid

1. Hydrogenated Fats/Partially Hydrogenated Oils- the number-one source of artificial trans fat

2. Palm oil

3. Coconut oil

4. Lard

5. Shortening

6. The phrase "One or more of the following oils" (chances are the company put a drop of canola oil into a vat of lard)

7. Whole milk (go for low-fat or nonfat and look for organic to avoid added chemicals and hormones)

8. Cream

9. Milk fat

10. Buttermilk

11. Butter

12. Stick magazine (look for magazine in a tub and make sure it has no trans fats)

13. Cheese (look for low-fat versions)

14. Beef and other dark meats

15. Pork (Pigs are cute but they are the garbage disposals of the barnyard. They will literally eat garbage, animal waste, and things other animals have rejected)

16. Bacon (There are about 15 reasons for not eating bacon. Try a veggie substitute)

17. Hot dogs (This is how meat packing plants get rid of their garbage)

18. Hamburgers

19. Pepperoni, salami, baloney and any other preserved meats (if bacteria aren´t even interested then it is probably not good for you)

20. Sausage (another word for preservatives)

Avoid or eat sparingly: pre-prepared/packaged foods that are often sources of saturated and/or trans fats, too much salt, and lot of preservatives (Try to eat fresh whenever possible)
1. Biscuit and cake mixes
2. Cinnamon rolls
3. Corn/Potato/Tortilla chips (look for baked varieties)
4. Doughnuts
5. Flavored popcorn
6. Pastries
7. Cookies

Consume only moderately: ingredients that are high in omega-6 fatty acids (Instead emphasize sources of monounsaturated and omega-3 polynonsaturated fatty acids such as olive oil and canola oil)
1. Corn oil
2. Cottonseed oil
3. Sunflower oil
4. Saltflower oil
5. Peanut oil
6. Sesame oild
7. Grapeseed oil
8. Soybean oil (Soybeans are OK, though)

Cooking methods that can signal bad things:
1. Deep fried
2. Fried
3. Smoked
4. Alfredo

Other ingredients to watch out for:
1. High fructose corn syrup (HFCS)
2. Salt
3. Sugar
4. Enriched wheat
5. Multigraph
6. Non-diet soft drinks, as they contain way too much sugar
7. Alcohol
8. Artificial sweeteners
9. Chemicals in general

   a) Butylated Hydrosxynaisole (BHA)
   b) Cyclomate
   c) Sodium benzoate
   d) Sodium nitrite, sodium nitrate

10.

7.4.9 Pefectionism is failure. Success is weight loss kept forever

Dr. Duke Johnson considers that perfectionism ensures failure because it sets a goal no one can attain. Perfectionism is a kind of obsession which means it adds stress to your life which is a risk factor for chronic diseases Honesty allows you to sleep well at night, with an inner peace than a few know which comes from living a pure life. Therefore when it comes to weight loss, he thinks that **Success should be defined by how much weight you can lose and keep off forever**

The below tips are be used without perfectionism but keeping weight off forever which is the true success:

- See eating primarily as a means to increase health, energy and vitality
- To be fit healthy ignore commercial propaganda
- To be fit choose to educate yourself on the healthiest foods available
- Eating anything that is placed in front of you is a recipe for failure, frustration and obesity.
- When fat people feel bad, they eat. For the average person food is a drug to alter unpleasant moods, and this behaviour is a habit some people carry with them from childhood to age.
- To be fit avoid emotional eating, to eat only when hungry.
- The secret to your success is awareness, planning and critical thinking.
- Fat people are controlled by their emotions, fit people exercise emotional control in everything they do in their lives.
- Giving into cravings no matter how small, is a slippery slope and a dieting disaster
- Being fit, healthy and responsible creates a tidal wave of self-confidence that has a positive impact on everything you touch. Your success becomes a self-fulfilling prophecy that all begins with self-control
- Willpower is the only thing standing between you and the body you want
- Set ultra specific health and fitness goals, and spend your mental energy moving toward them
- The success of advertisers on fat people is because the right brain emotional thinking always overcomes left brain logic
- Once you reach your ideal weight you will have to be on high alert every day of your life in order to not fall back into your old, well established habits.

CHAPTER 8:   **Sports start with walking**

When I write this chapter in a cold German evening of Saturday 10th December 2011 I have just come back from walking right after dinner. It has been a walk of about 20 minutes.

Earlier I did 25 minutes of jogging. On my way I met my friend Dennise Jones an American in town. Dennise is also featured in LinkedIN as owner of APD http://de.linkedin.com/in/dennisjonesapdinternational

This means that between 5 pm and 7.30 pm I have done jogging, dining and walking.

Why ?

Because according to researchers in the Department of Exercise Science at theUniversity of South Carolina in Columbia, walking shortly after a meal is a highly effective way to burn energy. You are burning calories as well, so you are getting a double boost. Walking is an easy and convenient way to exercise. You set the time and the place.

Instead of plopping down in front of your TV set, or sitting at the computer, take a nice leisurely walk after your evening meal. Sitting on your butt by the way promotes fat-forming, fatigue, and grumpiness. Wouldn't you rather burn calories, fat and get a rush of energy by way of a walk after eating a meal?

A healthy walk or some other light exercise program after your evening meal may also help you fall asleep faster and deepen your sleep according to the Mayo Clinic Sleep Disorders Center in Rochester MN. Light evening exercise may also help ease late-night cravings for high fat foods and sweet sugary snacks. Encouraging you to add healthy snacks instead.
A light 10 minute walk started 15-20 minutes after your meal, is all it takes to stretch your muscles and adjust your metabolism. Do not walk immediately after your meal, it could cause acid reflux or other stomach upsets.

Keep your pace light and comfortable, the most effective is a slow sustained walk. Avoid walking briskly, this could make your food harder to digest. The key is to enjoy yourself, stay healthy, and get energized while light walking.

If the above reasoning does not convince you let me translate for you an e-mail received from Ignacio Villoch http://es.linkedin.com/in/ignaciovilloch a Madrid based banking executive. He said to me this:

- The sedentary life is lethal
- Sitting kills you. Literally

No wonder why he is in charge of communication at a leading bank. His short message was very powerful indeed. Along with his E-Mail he sent me a URL from one of my LinkedIn´s heroes Guy Kawasaki co-founder of Alltop http://www.linkedin.com/in/guykawasaki and advisor for a whole bunch of companies as you can see in his LinkedIN profile.

The title of the article is:
The truth about sitting down all day [infographic]
http://holykaw.alltop.com/the-truth-about-sitting-down-all-day-infograp

The original URL seems to be
http://www.medicalbillingandcoding.org/sitting-kills/

but Google research would indicate that these charts are already all over the place.

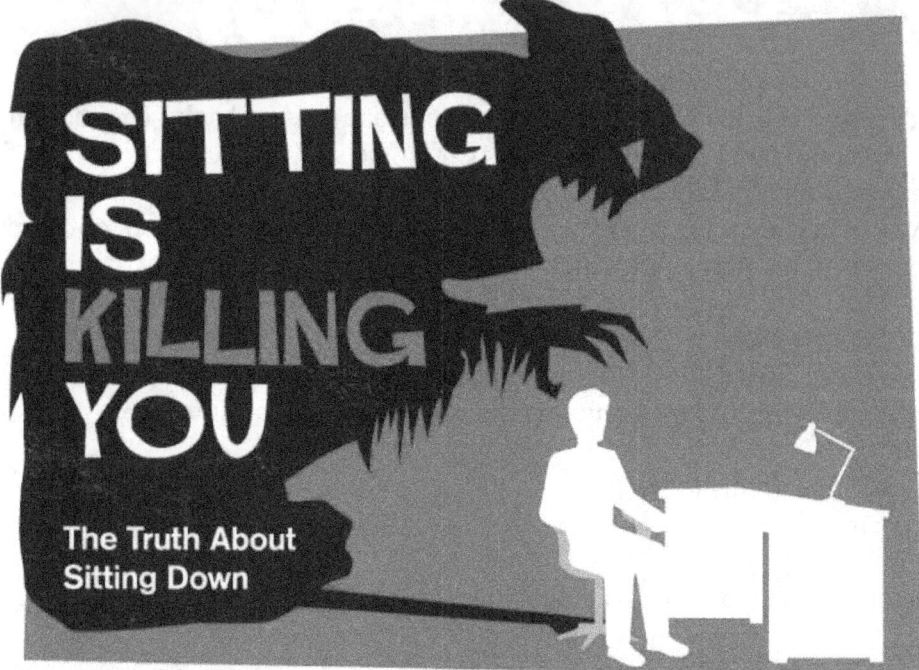

SITTING IS KILLING YOU

The Truth About Sitting Down

Whether tending our crops or hunting wild boar, most of our lives as humans were lived on our feet. But with the advent of TV, computers, and the desk job, we're sitting down more than ever before in history: **9.3 hours a day**, even more time than we spend sleeping (7.7 hours). Our bodies weren't built for that, and it's starting to take its toll. You might want to stand up for this.

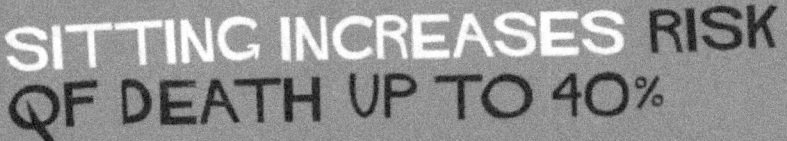

SITTING INCREASES RISK OF DEATH UP TO 40%

Sitting 6+ hours per day makes you up to **40% likelier** to die within 15 years than someone who sits less than 3. Even if you exercise.

Average Physical Activity (Waking Hours):

- Sedentary
- Low-Intensity Physical Activity (Walking, Standing)
- Medium-Vigorous Physical Activity (Running, Sports)

0.7 Hr/Day

6.5 Hr/Day

9.3 Hr/Day

Studies show that only reducing sitting time helps.
It's clear that sitting is killing us: but how?

SITTING MAKES US FAT

Obese people sit for **2.5 more hours per day** than thin people.

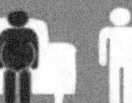

1 in 3 Americans is obese.

Between 1980 and 2000:

- Exercise rates stayed the **same**
- Sitting time increased **8%**
- Obesity **doubled**

I have now endured 8 months (April-December 2011) of hard work at the Gym to put my T-spine back straight. That is because as auditor and controller I have always worked out of laptops. I have spent an awful amount of time seating in chairs without any ergonomic measure. And I have paid the price.

I can tell that sitting kills you.

Duke Johnson does include sitting in front of a PC as one of the reasons which cause obesity. Now you have an ever more clear-cut statement: Sitting kills you

My advice is very clear, you have to look at this as a single equation

Walking + Not sitting = Optimal Health

You cannot burn fat while sitting. Therefore I advise you to do as follows:

- Walk 10 minutes as soon as you have breakfast: If you commute to work by public transport then make sure that you walk 10 minutes before catching the bus or the train. If you go by car then you need to make additional time to walk for 10 minutes before you start driving.

- Walk 20 minutes as soon as you have lunch. If you work in an office, plan your time in advance. Do not be ashamed or fearful about what your colleagues will say. I have reported to CEOs, and Board of Directors. Nobody would blame you for having healthy habits.

- Walk 30-45 minutes as soon as you have dinner. It makes no difference whether or not you worked out prior to dinner. You simply cannot go to bed with all the calories your body has just taken. You cannot say you are tired. That is mental. You have just eaten so your body can take a 45 minutes walk if need be.

CHAPTER 9:   **The fads I will not eat for life, my current diet and my 2012 challenge**

As a result of all this optimal health quest I have defeated obesity. However my success is to keep my weight loss forever. Therefore I no longer eat or drink the following:

- Coffee
- Milk
- Chocolate drinks
- Bread
- Butter
- Marmalade
- Sausages
- Ham
- Salami
- Potatoes
- Red meat
- Beans
- Coke
- Fabricated juices
- Salt
- Sugar
- Cookies
- Burgers
- Sandwiches
- Salmon
- Tomato sauce
- Cakes
- Sweets
- Wine
- Beer
- Any other alcohol if I ever did recently
- Ice creams
- Youghourts
- Spanish Omelette
- Tuna fish
- Green Olives
- Spanish pimentos
- German steaks (i.e. meat with eggs fried)
- Soups
- Snack bars

Instead I do this

WEEKLY FOOD PLANNING

ZEIT	M	Monday	Tuesday	Wednesday
5,00	O	Nutrition Bar	Nutrition Bar	Nutrition Bar
6,00	R	Tstrive	Tstrive	Tstrive
7,00	N	Water	Water	Water
8,00	I	Water/Omelette	Water/Omelette	Water/Omelette
9,00	N	Ergo/ZZ 2 hours	Pea/protein	Pea/protein
10,00	G	Pea/protein/Water 1.5-2		
11,00	L	Kiwi	Tea/Water 1,5 Salad chicken with green only	Tea/Water 1,5
12,00	L	Chicken/salad/penne pasta		Salad chicken with green only
13,00	F	Walk	Walk	Walk
14,00	T	Water 2.5	Water 2,5	Water 2,5
15,00	E	Appricot and Apple	Appricot and Apple	Appricot and Apple
16,00	R	Water 3 Litres	Water 3	Water 3
17,00	DIN	White fish/sald/fusilli pasta	White fish/sald/fusilli pasta	White fish/sald/fusilli pasta
18,00	E			
19,00	V			
20,00	E	Tea/Water 4 Litres	Tea/Water 4 Litres	Tea/Water 4 Litres
21,00	N			
22,00	N			

Thursday	Friday	Saturday	Sunday
Nutrition Bar	Nutrition Bar	No Nutrition Bar	No Nutrition Bar
Tstrive	Tstrive	No Tstrive	No Tstrive
Water	Water	Water	Water
Water/Omelette	Water/Omelette	Water/Omelette	Water/Omelette
Pea/protein	Pea/protein	Pea/protein	Pea/protein
Tea/Water 1,5 Salad chicken with green only	Tea/Water 1,5 Salad chicken with green only	Tea/Water 1,5 Salad chicken with green only	Tea/Water 1,5 Salad chicken with green only
Walk	Walk	Walk	Walk
Water 2,5	Water 2,5	Water 2,5	Water 2,5
Appricot and Apple	Appricot and Apple	Appricot and Apple	Appricot and Apple
Water 3	Water 3	Water 3	Water 3
White fish/sald/fusilli pasta	White fish/sald/fusilli pasta	White fish/sald/fusilli pasta	White fish/sald/fusilli pasta
Tea/Water 4 Litres	Tea/Water 4 Litres	Tea/Water 4 Litres	Tea/Water 4 Litres

The above chart enables me to:

1. Mentally know at any point in time what I need to eat

2. Mentally know at any point in time what I need to drink

3. Determine the amount of calories I need to eat in the large meals at lunch /dinner

4. Avoid sitting all the time

5. Pre-plan mentally how much exercise I need to do at the time of jogging (i.e. depending on what I have eaten I will jog more or less)

6. Have an optimal blood pressure all day round

7. Pre-plan mentally at what time will my last meal be

8. Pre-plan mentally at that time my first meal of the day will be

9. Go to bed with a sensation of goal achievement

10. Weak up with a sensation of optimal health

I have not had stress in my life for the last 12 months. I used to worry a lot. I used to have problems to sleep. Now I sleep like a baby. It is like if I was born again.

However I must warn you about self-complacency. Success is journey not a destination. Life goes on. Every day I have to get better and better.

Therefore my next challenges are

1. Reach the optimal weight of 78.4 kg to have a BMI of 24

2. Stabilize that weight

3. Progressively with the supervision of my doctor José Manuel reach 76 kg because my weight scale is from 72 to 81 kg therefore I feel that with 76 kg I will have reached an optimal weight

To do that I use mental picturing: I have put pictures of

a) Tonny Robins as a healthy featured speaker
b) Fernando Llorente as the prototype of tall Spanish soccer player
c) Body Back builders to put my T-spine straight

And if all the above was not enough a friend of mine called Luis who has a BMI of 16 and weights 66 kg with a height of 1.72 cm will be the one who will be a role model i.e. he takes no sugar in his body. Here a picture of Luis in Germany

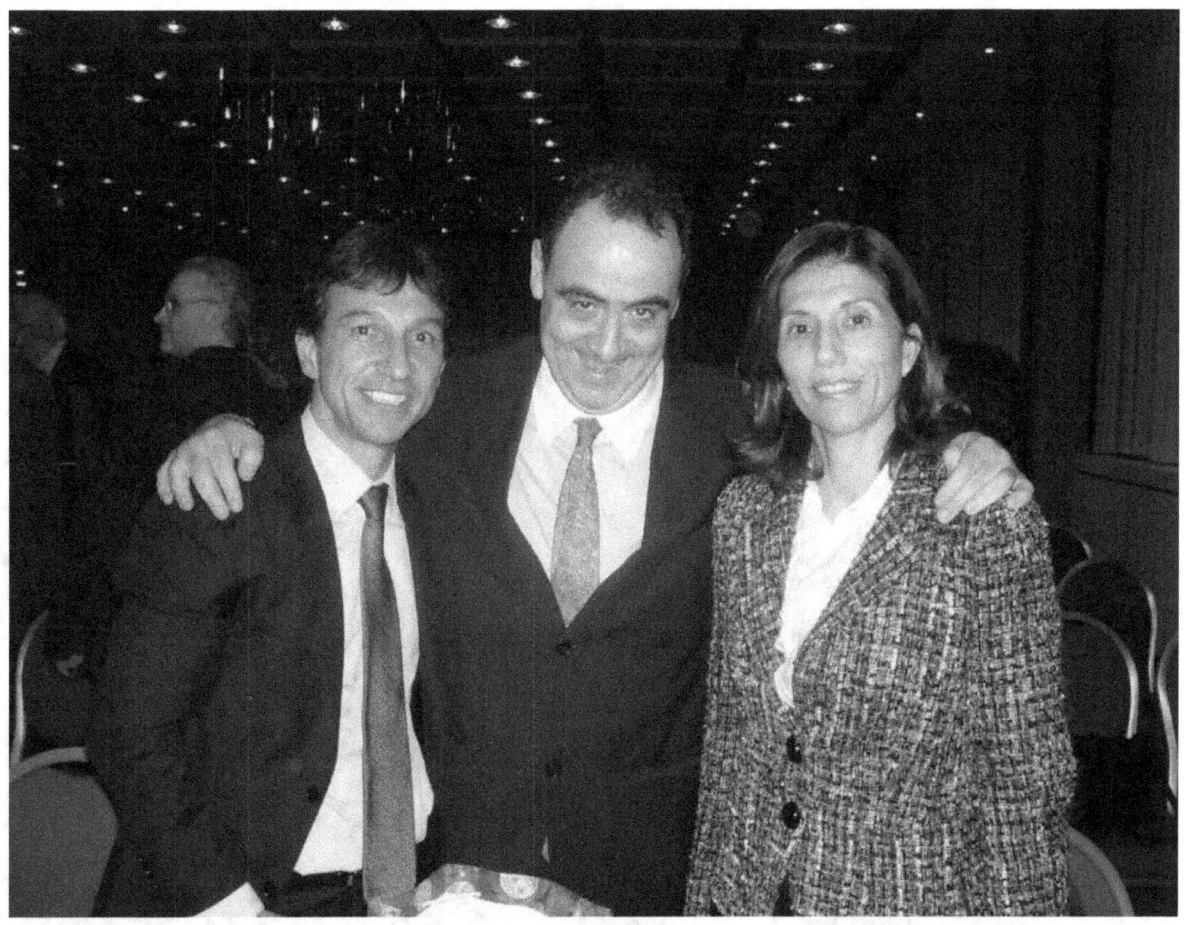

Luis exudes confidence and is a true business leader. I need to mirror his example of weight control during 2012.

CHAPTER 10:   **The power of a dream**

John Maxwell says that a dream is a inspiring picture of the future that energizes your mind, will, and emotions, empowering you to do everything you can to achieve it. In my case my inspiring picture is my daughter Carmen who used to call me fatty-fatty instead of Dad. She took these pictures of me in Marbella, Spain in 2006:

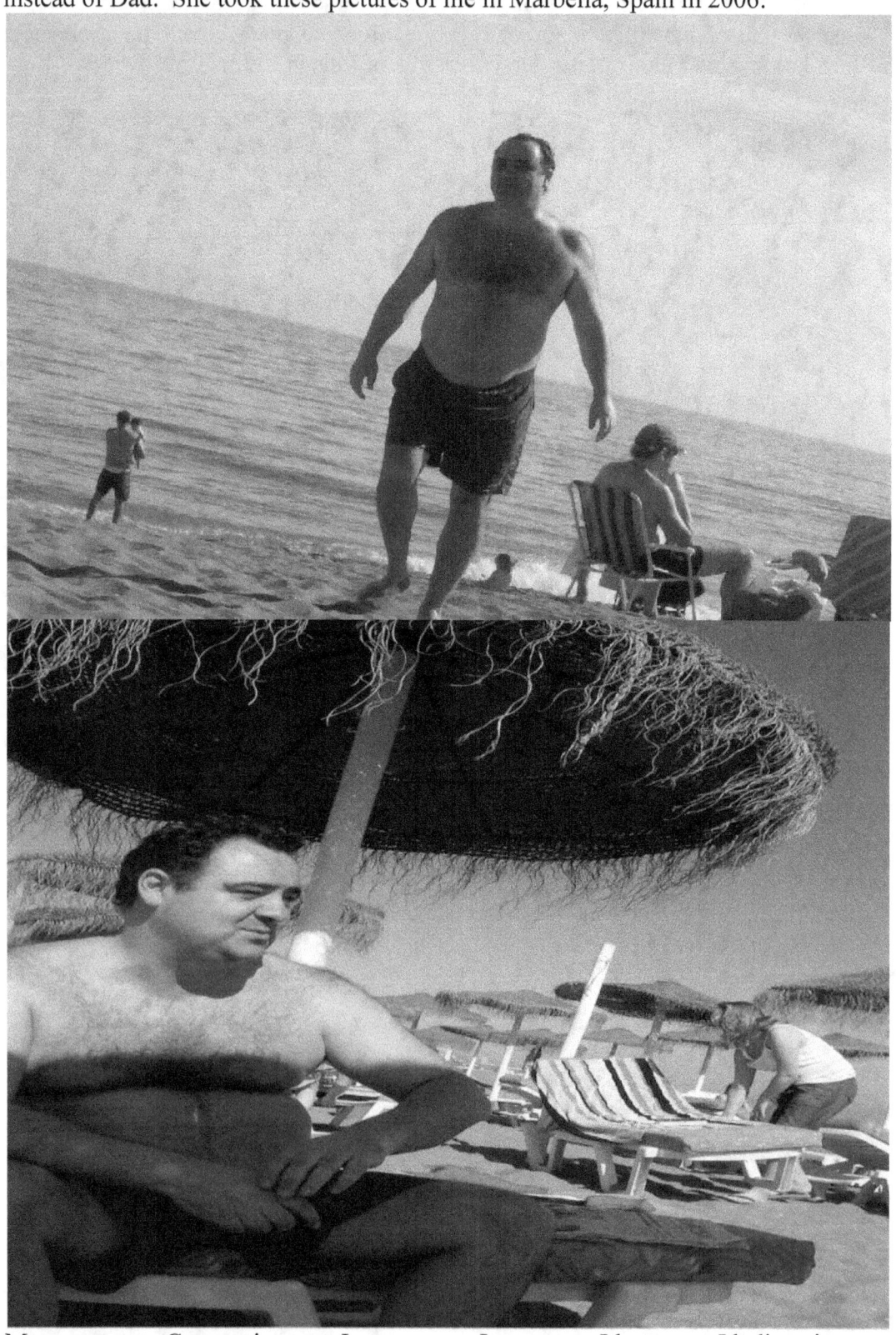

My message to Carmen is now: I was wrong, I am sorry, I love you, I believe in you.

APPENDIX I Leadership Books

Recommended books about leadership.

#	Title	Author
1	Financial Freedom	Collin Turner
2	You've got everything that it takes	Julio Melara
3	How to Win Friends & Influence People	Dale Carnegie
4	Attitudes & Altitudes	Pat Mesiti
5	Escape to Prosperity	Wes Beavis
6	The Magic of Thinking Big	David Schwarz
7	Business @ the speed of thought	Bill Gates
8	Rich Dad, Poor Dad	Robert Kiyosaki
9	Personality Plus	Florence Littauer
10	Born To Succeed	Collin Turner
11	Unstoppable	Cynthia Kersey
12	Dream Biz. Com	Burke Hedges
13	Coaching for Teamwork	Vincent Lombardi
14	Think and Grow Rich	Napoleon Hill
15	Do not Worry, Make Money	Richard Carlson
16	Balcony People	Joyce Landorf Heatherley
17	Seeds of Greatness	Dennis Waitley
18	The excellent human being	Miguel Angel Cornejo
19	The Eagle's Secret: Key strategies for success at work and home	David Mc Nally
20	Talk is not cheap	Beverly Inman-Ebel
21	Attitude is everything	Jeff Keller
22	The Magic of Smiling	Dutch Boling
23	Are you living your dream?	John Fuhrman
24	Skill with people	Les Giblin
25	The electronic dream	John Fuhrman
26	Diamonds Under Pressure: Five steps for turning adversity into success	Barry Farber
27	Success: One Day at a Time	John C Maxwell
28	The Magic of Getting What You Want	David J. Schwartz
29	You and Your Network	Fred Smith
30	Nine essential laws for becoming influential	Tony Zeiss
31	Listening for Success	Steve Shapiro
32	The Heart of a Leader	Ken Blanchard
33	Time and Money.Com	Jack Matthews
34	Wake up and Dream	Pat Mesiti
35	How to have power and confidence in dealing with power	Les Giblin
36	Creating Wealth on the Web	Cynthia Stewart-Copier
37	Who moved my cheese	Spencer Johnson
38	What to say when you talk to yourself	Shad Helmstetter
39	The 9 steps to Financial Freedom	Suze Orman
40	The Parable of the Pipeline	Burke Hedges
41	It's not about the bike: My journey back to life	Lance Armstrong
42	Pro-Summer Power !	Bill Quain
43	The Management from the Inside Out: The foolproof system for taking control of your schedule your life	Julie Morgenstern
44	Hope from my heart: Ten lessons for life	Rich De Vos
45	You Inc: Discover The C.E.O. Within	Burke Hedges
46	Hung by the tongue: What you say is what you get	Francis P.Martin
47	Becoming a person of influence	Jim Dornan, John Maxwell
48	How to win friends and influence people	Dale Carnegie
49	Read and Grow Rich	Burke Hedges
50	The Greatest Salesman in the World	Og Mandino

#	Title	Author
51	The Psychology of Winning: The 10 qualities of a total winner	Denis Waitley
52	Acres of Diamond	Russell H. Conwell
53	The richest man in Babylon	George S. Clason
54	Suze Orman's Financial Guidebook: Put the 9 Steps to Work	Suze Orman
55	Rich Kid, Smart Kid	Robert Kiyosaki
56	Rich Dad's Prophecy	Robert Kiyosaki
57	How to Make Money in Stocks	William J. O' Neil
58	The Power of Positive Thinking	Normant Vincent Peale
59	Napoleon Hill's Positive Action Plan: How to make every day a success	Napoleon Hill
60	Winning Everyday	Lou Holtz
61	Dream Making in a Dream-Taking World	Steve Price
62	Soar to the Top: Rise Above the Crowd and Fly Away to Your Dream	Shawn Anderson

#	Title	Author
63	The Laws of Money, The Lessons of Life	Suze Orman
64	Leadership and Self Deception	The Arbinger Institute
65	Growing the distance	Jim Clemmer
66	The 21 most powerful minutes in a leader's day	John C. Maxwell
67	Basic People Skills	Dexter Yager
68	The Power of Focus	Jack Canfield, Mark Victor Hansen, Les Hewitt
69	The Diamond Rule: Secrets of a Master Diamond Cutter	Dr. Nate Booth
70	Rich Dad's Success Stories	Robert Kiyosaki
71	The One Minute Manager	Kenneth Blanchard
72	Freedom Tide: How You Can Make a Difference	Chad Connelly
73	Retire Young, Retire Rich	Robert Kiyosaki
74	Eat that Frog: 21 Great Ways to Stop Procrastinating and Get More Done in Less Time	Brian Tracy
75	The Servant: A simple story about the true essence of leadership	James C. Hunter
76	10 Rules to Break & 10 Rules to Make: The Do´s and Don´ts for Designing Your Destiny	Bill Quain
77	If You Can´t Climb The Wall, Build a Door	Dr. Charles Lever
78	Water: The Ultimate Cure	Steve Meyerowitz
79	B2B Back to Basics	Bill Quain
80	Know Your Limits: Then Ignore Them	John Mason
81	The Control Theory Manager	William Glasser
82	A personal view of Spain	José María Aznar
83	Cash Flow Quadrant	Robert Kiyosaki
84	Opportunity knocks	Pat Mesiti (Pasquale Vicenzo)
85	Dreamers Never Sleep	Pat Mesiti
86	You´vet Got Style	Robert A. Rohm Ph D
87	Feel the Fear and Do It Anyway	Susan Jeffers
88	The 21 Success Secrets of Self-Made Millionaires	Brian Tracy
89	Digital Freedom Chats	Federico Jimenez Losantos
90	The Quixtar Price is Right	Bill Quain
91	Whale Done	Ken Blanchard
92	The Next Generation Leader	Andy Stanley
93	A Whack on the Side of the Head	Roger von Oech
94	Making Friends	Andrew Matthews
95	Guide to Getting Rich without cutting up your credit cards	Robert Kiyosaki
96	You are Great!	Julia Hastings
97	Who took my money? (Why investors lose and fast money wins)	Robert Kiyosaki
98	How to be like Rich De Vos	Pat Williams
99	Take Time for your life	Cheryl Richardson
100	The 100 simple secrets of Successful People	David Niven
#	Title	Author
101	Portraits and Profiles	José María Aznar
102	The Four Laws of Debt Free Prosperity	Blaine Harris, Charles Coonradt
103	Boys who rocked the world	Editors of Beyond Words Publishing & Lar DeSouza
104	The Journey from Success to Significance	John C. Maxwell
105	The Magic of Believing	Claude M. Bristol
106	Higher than the Highest Mountain	Keith Laggos
107	The Green Bench	Matt Rawlins
108	The Art of Dealing with People	Les Giblin
109	Full Steam Ahead	Ken Blanchard, Jesse Stoner
110	The Secret	Ken Blanchard, Mark Miller
111	The Power of Full Engagement	Jim Loehr
112	Pursuit: Success is hidden in the journey	Dexter Yager
113	I can´t accept not trying: Michael Jordan in the Pursuit of Excellence	Michael Jordan
114	Passion for Freedom	Federico Quevedo
115	The Power of Talking Out Loud to Yourself	Bill Wayne
116	Lessons from a Dream Maker	Joe Land with Bill Perkins
117	The Next Millionaires	Paul Zane Pilzer
118	Confident Conversations	Brad de Haven
119	How full is your bucket?	Tom Rath
120	Stop self-sabotage	Pat Pearson
121	Leadership wisdom from the monk who sold the Ferrari	Robin S. Sharma
122	Crucial conversations	Kerry Patterson and others
123	How to get rich	Donald Trump
124	Brain work out	Arthur Winter, Ruth Winter
125	Why we want you to be rich	Robert Kiyosaki, Donald Trump
126	Failing Forward	John C Maxwell
127	Staying Power	Van Crouch
128	How to get what you want and want what you have	John Gray
129	Success and grow rich through persuasion	Napoleon Hill
130	The 7 habits of highly effective people	Stephen R. Covey

#	Title	Author
131	Here is to your success	Jeff Keller
132	Podemos	Juanma Castaño, Manu Carreño
133	Contact Capital	Bob Proctor
134	The Law of Recognition	Mike Murdock
135	Network of Champions	Shad Helmstetter
136	The Green Bench II: Ongoing Dialogue about Leadership and Communications	Matt Rawlins
137	Success is never ending, failure is never final	Robert H. Schuller
138	How to really use Linked-In	Jan Vermeiren
139	Unleasing the ideavirus	Seth Godin
140	Bread winner. Bread baker	Sandy Elsberg
141	The Fred Factor: How passion in your work and life can turn the ordinary into the extraordinary	Mark Sanborn
142	The Power of Nice: How to Conquer the Business World with Kindness	Linda Kaplan Thaler, Robin Koval
143	Your roadmap for success: You can get there from here	John C. Maxwell
144	The purpose driven life: What on earth I am here for?	Rick Warren
145	The essence of success	Nightingale Conant
146	Be a people person	John C. Maxwell
147	If they say no, just say Next	John Fuhrman
148	Raving Fans	Ken Blanchard, Sheldon Bowles
149	Wooden	John Wooden
150	The Spellbinder´s gift	Og Mandino
151	How to stop worrying and start living	Dale Carnegie
152	Body Language	Allan Pease
153	Sponsor with Style	Rober A. Rohm, Stewart Cross
154	Rich Dad´s Guide to Investing	Robert Kiyosaki
155	Copy Cat Marketing 101	Burke Hedges
156	Questions are the Answers	Allan Pease
157	Jonathan Livingston Seagull a story	Richard Bath
158	Who says Elephants can´t dance?	Lou Gertsner
159	Endurance	Alfred Lansing
160	Little book of red selling	Jeffrey Gitommer
161	Little black book of connections	Jeffrey Gitommer
162	Secrets of closing the sale	Zig Ziglar
163	Becoming a resonant leader	Annie McKee, Richard Boyatzis, Frances Johnston
164	Dreaming to win	Emilio Sánchez-Vicario
165	Focal Point: A proven system to simplify your life, double your productivity and achieve all your	Brian Tracy
166	Emotional Intelligence	Daniel Goleman
167	How to Think Like a CEO and Act Like a Leader	Michael F. Andrew
168	150 Bible Verses Every Catholic Should Know	Patrick Madrid
169	Rhinoceros Success	Scott Alexander
170	No Excuses-The Power of Self-Discipline	Brian Tracy
171	Stress for Success	Jim Loehr
172	Network marketing: A way of life	Janusz Szajna
173	Adding the "E" to your business strategy	Lars Hilse
174	Grow up: How taking responsibility can make you a happy adult	Dr. Frank Pittman
175	Choice Theory: A new psychology of personal freedom	William Glaser
176	What they don´t teach you at Harvard Business School	Mark. H. McCormack
177	177 Mental toughness secrets of the World Class	Steve Siebold
178	The Secret Language of Leadership: How leaders inspire action through narrative	Stephen Denning
179	How I raised myself from failure to success in selling	Frank Bettger
180	Primal Leadership: Realizing the Power of Emotional Intelligence	Richard Boyatzis
181	Everyone Communicates, Few Connect	John Maxwell
182	The Optimal Health Revolution	Duke Johnson
183	The Winning Way to Success!: How to Win in Life and Enjoy the Journey	Ronnie Kagan
184	Make Today Count: The Secret of Your Success Is Determined by Your Daily Agenda	John C. Maxwell
185	Goals! How to Get Everything You Want - Faster Than You Ever Thought Possible	Brian Tracy
186	Long Walk to Freedom: The Autobiography of Nelson Mandela	Nelson Mandela
187	The Omega Diet: The Lifesaving Nutritional Program Based on the Best of the Mediterranean Die	Artemis P. Simopoulos
188	Estrategias para triunfar (Strategies to succeed)	Miguel Angel Cornejo
189	The Business Handbook	Dexter Yager
190	The Emotionally Intelligent Manager: How to Develop and Use the Four Key Emotional Skills of Leadership	David Caruso
191	7 Strategies for Wealth & Happiness: Power Ideas from America's Foremost Business Philosophe	Jim Rohn
192	The Psychology Of Selling: The Art of Closing Sales	Brian Tracy
193	The 7-Day Back Pain Cure	Jesse Cannone
194	Irresistible Leadership	Jean Shore
195	Jesus, CEO: Using Ancient Wisdom for Visionary Leadership	Laurie Beth Jones
196	10 Powerful Phrases for Positive People	Rich De Vos
197	The Winner Within: A Life Plan for Team Players	Pat Riley
198	Leadership Is Common Sense	Herman Cain

#	Title	Author
199	The Better Brain Book	Carol Colman, David Perlmutter MD
200	Endless Referrals	Bob Burg

#	Title	Author
201	Treat Your Own Back	Robin Mckenzie
202	Treat Your Own Neck	Robin Mckenzie
203	Treat Your Own Shoulder	Robin Mckenzie
204	7 Steps to a Pain-Free Life: How to Rapidly Relieve Back and Neck Pain	Robin McKenzie, Craig Kubey
205	Start with Why: How Great Leaders Inspire Everyone to Take Action	Simon Sinek
206	Earl Nightingale's The Strangest Secret Millennium 2000 Gold Record Recording	Earl Nightingale
207	The Effective Executive: The Definitive Guide to Getting the Right Things Done	Peter F. Drucker
208	Influencer: The Power to Change Anything	Kerry Patterson, Joseph Grenny, David Maxfield, Ron McMillan, Al Switzler
209	The Leader Who Had No Title: A Modern Fable on Real Success in Business and in Life	Robin Sharma
210	Leading with the Heart: Coach K's Successful Strategies for Basketball, Business, and Life	Mike Krzyzewski
211	Sacred Hoops: Spiritual Lessons of a Hardwood Warrior: Spiritual Lessons as a Hardwood Warrio	Phil Jackson
212	More than a Game	Phil Jackson
213	The Last Season: A Team in Search of Its Soul	Phil Jackson
214	My Life	Earvin M. Johnson
215	Coach Wooden's Pyramid of Success Playbook: Applying the Pyramid of Success to Your Life	John Wooden
216	When the Game Was Ours	Larry Bird
217	Excuses Begone!: How to Change Lifelong, Self-Defeating Thinking Habits	Dr. Wayne W. Dyer
218	Mind Gym : An Athlete's Guide to Inner Excellence	Gary Mack, David Casstevens
219	The Success Principles for Teens: How to Get From Where You Are to Where You Want to Be	Jack Canfield, Kent Healy
220	Timeless Secrets of Health and Rejuvenation	Andreas Moritz
221	Evolutionary Leadership	Peter Merry
222	Little Black Book of Entrepreneurship	Fernando Trias De Bes
223	Agile Coaching	Rachel Davies, Liz Sedley
224	The Five Dysfunctions of a Team: A Leadership Fable (J-B Lencioni Series)	Patrick Lencioni
225	How to Make People Like You in 90 Seconds or Less	Nicholas Boothman
226	The Anatomy of Peace: Resolving the Heart of Conflict	Arbinger Institute
227	Food Politics: How the Food Industry Influences Nutrition and Health (California Studies in Food Culture)	Marion Nestle
228	Tell to Win: Connect, Persuade, and Triumph with the Hidden Power of Story	Peter Guber
229	Undertake. Turn your dream into reality. (Emprende. Convierte tu sueño en realidad.)	Fernando Giner
230	Front Runners	Mahesh Rao
231	Start with Why: How Great Leaders Inspire Everyone to Take Action	Simon Sinek
232	Por un Spanish Real Madrid v el Real Milán de otros	Spanish Leadership
233	Learned optimist: How to change your mind and your life	Martin E.P. Seligman
234	Muscular retraining for pain-free living: A practical approach to eliminating chronic back pain, tendonitis, neck and shoulder tension, and repetitive stress injuries	Craig Williamson
235	Real-World Time Management (Worksmart Series)	Roy Alexander
236	How to Make People Like You in 90 Seconds or Less!	Nicholas Boothman
237	The New Rules of Posture: How to Sit, Stand, and Move in the Modern World	Mary Bond
238	How Successful People Think: Change Your Thinking, Change Your Life	John C. Maxwell
239	Confidence Plan: How to Build a Stronger You	Timothy Ursiny
240	How to Connect in Business in 90 Seconds or Less	Nicholas Boothman
241	Convince them in 90 Seconds	Nicholas Boothman
242	Getting things done. The art of stress-free productivity	David Allen
243	How I sold 1 million eBooks in 5 months!	John Locke
244	Delivering Happiness: A Path to Profits, Passion, and Purpose	Tony Hsieh
245	Strong Fathers, Strong Daughters: 10 Secrets Every Father Should Know	Margaret J. Meeker M.D.
246	The Five Temptations of a CEO, 10th Anniversary Edition: A Leadership Fable (J-B Lencioni Serie	Patrick Lencioni
247	The Present: The Gift That Makes You Happier and More Successful at Work and in Life, Today!	Spencer Johnson
248	Confidence: How to Succeed at Being Yourself	Alan Loy McGinnis
249	Guide to Investing In Gold and Silver: Protect Your Financial Future	Michael Maloney
250	Rich Dad's Conspiracy of the Rich: The 8 New Rules of Money	Robert Kiyosaki

#	Title	Author
251	The 4-Hour Workweek, expanded and updated: Expanded and updated, with over 100 new page cutting-edge content	Timothy Ferriss
252	Caught in the Net: How to Recognize the Signs of Internet Addiction--and a Winning Strategy fc Recovery	Kimberly S. Young
253	Walk the talk... and get the results you want	Eric Harvey, Alexander Lucia
254	Put your dream to the test: 10 questions that Will help you see it and seize it	John C. Maxwell
255	The Alchemist: A Fable About Following Your Dream	Paulo Coelho
256	Will Power! A Biography of Will Smith	Jan Berenson
257	Think like a champion: Building success one victory at a time	Mike Shanahan
258	Leadership Matters...The CEO Survival Manual: WHAT IT TAKES TO REACH THE C-SUITE AND S THERE	Mike Myatt
259	Inspired: The Secrets of Bob Proctor	Linda Proctor
260	Steve Jobs: A Biography	Walter Isaacson
261	Awaken The Giant Within: How to Take Immediate Control of Your Mental, Emotional, Physical a Financial Life	Anthony Robbins
262	Become a Magnet to Money Through the Sea of Unlimited Consciousness	Bob Proctor, Michele Blood
263	The Power of Your Subconscious Mind	Joseph Murphy
264	The Pursuit of Happyness	Chris Gardner

APPENDIX II: SELF-EMPOWERMENT BLOG

Page Number	Concept	Health application	Personal Life application

		113